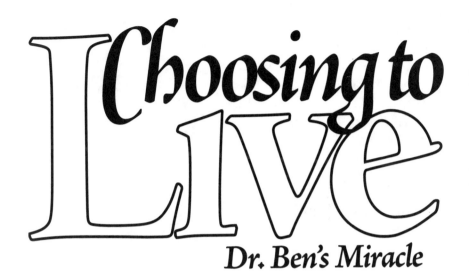

# Choosing to Live
## Dr. Ben's Miracle

# TRIUMPH OVER
# TERMINAL CANCER

By

Benjamin R. Sanidad, Jr., M.D.
with
Cecil Murphey

Printed By
Remnant Publications

**Choosing To Live**

This edition published 2002

Cover Design by Mark Bond

ISBN  0-9720982-0-8

# Choosing to Live

## Triumph Over Terminal Cancer

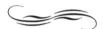

*For Additional Copies of this Book*
*Contact: Gayle Holback*
*P.O. Box 34*
*Marion, Ohio  43301-0034 U.S.A.*

*Phone: 740-383-2478*
*e-mail:* **info@choosingtolive.net**

# Thank You

to

The following friends who made this book possible by sharing their know-how and encouragements:

*Cecil Murphey, Becki Trueblood, Darlene Slack, Dr. Elma Lou Roda and Emmeline "Fraulein" Flores.*

To my doctors, nurses, hospital personnel, relatives and different Denominations of the Marion, Ohio community who cared and prayed for me.

# Special THANKS

to

*Gary and Gayle Holback*

Without your support this book would not have been printed.

*Mark Bond*

Designer of book cover (donated).

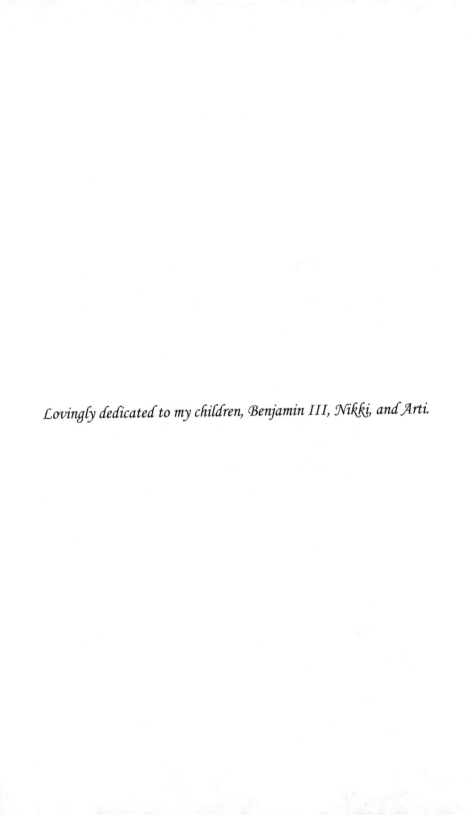

*Lovingly dedicated to my children, Benjamin III, Nikki, and Arti.*

# Contents

# Preface

After receiving the devastating news that I have cancer of the esophagus, I experienced many difficult trials, physically and emotionally. Like others who have had cancer before me, I faced physical pain and suffering, job loss, financial difficulties, fear, depression, and feelings of rejection. Why then would I want to relive these painful experiences by writing this book?

After beating the odds and surviving this disease, I decided to write this book in behalf of the numerous people who have approached me and wanted to know why I am alive today. This book will explain, in simple terms, the lifestyle changes that I have adopted to help prevent the spread of cancer. As a doctor, I made a radical decision when I chose to forego chemotherapy or radiation and commit myself to an alternative treatment program. My hope is that my experience will help others, especially those who may be diagnosed with cancer and other diseases. But although the lifestyle and treatment I chose worked for me, it is important to note that they might not work for everyone.

My experience is not unique. Many have experienced life-threatening situations and survived. It takes hard work and it also takes faith. Miracle? Yes, I believe my survival is a miracle. I am healthier than before. I have reassessed my priorities in life. I am closer to my wife and children. I have a deepened sensitivity to my patients because now I know the fears and questions they have. I am closer to God and am committed to doing God's work in the world. This book is a part of that service.

I also wrote this book to honor God who gave me another lease on my life and to give tribute to people who prayed for me and shared the pain and suffering that my family endured.

I hope and pray that this book will inspire you all and help you conquer cancer and other diseases, in quest of a better and more productive life.

In God's Love,
Ben

# Foreword

*by: Dr. Frederick Winegarner, General & vascular surgeon.*
*Physician of the Year 2001 Marion, OH.*

I came to Marion, Ohio from Indianapolis in 1978 and began a practice of general and vascular surgery. Dr. Benjamin Sanidad, Jr. was one of the anesthesiologists at Marion General Hospital and had the reputation of being an extremely competent anesthesiologist, was respected and well liked by his colleagues. Over the years, he administered anesthetics for many of my patients, some of whom were critical and in life threatening situations. On many occasions, we individually prayed for these patients in the operating room and through that developed a friendship bond that is not easily broken.

Over the years, I have had the privilege of providing medical care to other members of Dr. Sanidad's family. In late March of 1996, Dr. Sanidad was administering an anesthetic on a Saturday afternoon when he became very faint and was admitted to the hospital. On the following day, I examined his stomach and esophagus with a light and found a cancer in his esophagus. He was sent to Ohio State University where a total removal of his esophagus was done in an attempt to remove the tumor. There were two positive lymph nodes found outside the esophagus in the upper part of the abdominal cavity. This usually indicates a very poor long-term prognosis. It was expected that the tumor would return.

At that point, Dr. Sanidad had to make the decision between taking chemotherapy and/or radiation therapy or doing nothing. At that point, I believe he really heard from the Lord and made the decision to go a different route. He enrolled himself in a program, which only he can describe in detail; however, it involved changes in diet, exercise, sunlight and water treatment. He lost a considerable amount of weight but through this episode, he remained steadfastly healthy and free of any recurrence of the tumor.

Statistically, it was expected that his survival would only be eight months from the time of his surgery in April of 1996. Dr.

Sanidad turned his heart to the Lord and this was obvious to those who knew him personally. He was quick to give God the credit for his return to health. His return was not easy or spontaneous; it was gradual and steady. He has made a really remarkable recovery.

In October of 1997 while he was in Canada visiting with family, Dr. Sanidad became acutely ill and was taken to surgery by the physician in Canada. At that time, it was found that almost all of his small intestines was dusky colored and without adequate circulation. The bowel was observed, warmed up and seemed to improve. He was then taken back to surgery the following day for another look to be sure the bowel had remained alive and miraculously, he recovered from this without losing an inch of his intestines. This in itself is a real miracle as was his original recovery from the esophageal cancer.

Ben has continued to walk with the Lord, as has his family who has been extremely supportive and encouraging to Ben and also to those of us who have cared for Ben medically. They have also been supportive of those who have been friends of the family. His family have not only "talked the talk" with the Lord but they have actually "walked the walk" with the Lord. Ben and his wife have given an uplifting witness to each other, to their family, their neighbors and to all of those that know them. They continue to minister in service of the Lord. From my perspective, they have been faithful servants of the Lord, Jesus Christ. I am privileged to know them and to have been able to witness not one, but at least two miracles in his life. I wish him continued good health and an increasing closeness with the Lord Jesus Christ.

# The Shocking News

*"Yea, though I walk through the valley of the shadow of death,
I will fear no evil; for thou art with me."*
—Psalms 23:4 (KJV)

"Jim, I'm not feeling well."

Those unfamiliar words, spoken by me as an anesthesiologist in an operating room, began a series of events that would take me to the place of death twice in the next eighteen months.

"I'm not feeling well," sounds so simple, almost unimportant. Yet soon after I tried to dismiss their significance, the words took on a powerful meaning.

Ten minutes into an emergency gall bladder surgery, a sudden weakness swept over me. At first, I assumed it would go away, so I ignored it. But within minutes the exhaustion was so strong I felt as if I could not stand up any longer. My patient was asleep on the automatic ventilator, so I lay my head on my anesthesia chair and closed my eyes. I willed the weakness to go away, but it did not lessen. I lifted my head and looked around. Just then I saw everything in doubles. Instead of one light overhead, I saw two. Two patients. Two of everything I focused on. To a doctor, that was a clear indication that something was seriously wrong.

Too tired even to sit, I could feel myself sinking to the floor.

"Get the ER doctor," Dr. James Hering commanded the circulating nurse.

Because I obviously could not continue, they asked Dr. Madia, another anesthesiologist to come in. Meanwhile, Dr. Delos Reyes, the other anesthesiologist who was working in the operating room next to mine, ran back and forth caring for his own patient and mine.

Although aware of what was going on, the tiredness would not allow me even to speak. I wanted to go into a deep, deep sleep.

"Heart attack," I heard someone whisper. I had the obvious symptoms.

"Oh no, it can't be," I thought. "Not me." Even as I rejected those words, I knew it was possible. I was overweight, did not exercise regularly, and ate carelessly. I was also 51, which made me a good age for cardiac problems to appear.

Only that Saturday morning, March 30, 1996, four days after my birthday, I had mentioned to my wife, Esther, that I was not feeling especially well—nothing serious—just a sense of not being at my best. I did have a little bleeding in my mouth, but we assumed it was from my gums after brushing my teeth.

I had scheduled myself to be on second call—that is, I backed up one of our team of five anesthesiologists. He was fully booked already. Just as Esther was preparing to go to church, I received a call.

"Dr. Sanidad, we have an emergency Cesarean section," the operator said. "They need you to come in."

I rushed to the hospital, gulped down a cup of coffee and doughnut, and then prepared my patient for surgery. After that surgery, we had two more patients for labor epidural catheter insertion, followed by a hip operation. In the middle of a full morning, I drank another cup of coffee and ate two more doughnuts. The food made me feel a little better. On my way home at 2 p.m., the beeper paged me to return for an emergency gall bladder surgery. As soon as I reached the hospital, I wolfed down a hamburger and a coke in the cafeteria before rushing to surgery. That vague "not feeling well," did not prepare me for the humbling and disturbing experience of a doctor collapsing in surgery.

Two people, one on either side of me, lifted my arms. Right then I was too tired to open my eyes and see who they were. I did not care about anything, only resting. I felt my body being lifted from the cold floor.

"Walk slowly," said a muffled voice.

At first I thought, "I can't walk. I can't even stand up." After taking a couple of deep breaths, I opened my eyes and realized I was standing up. I took two steps, but my legs felt rubbery, weak, as if I had no control over them. The two people still held me and somehow my feet moved forward in a kind of dream-like state. They stayed with me until we reached the recovery room. Their arms held me up and I felt as if they were almost carrying me. It seemed like a long time before they helped me climb on to a gurney and lie down. I may have passed out, because I am not clear what happened next.

The next thing I remember was a doctor examining me. His cool hand touched my wrist and he opened the top of my shirt. I wanted to protest that I was all right, but I felt too weak to say a word. After he examined me and I lay quietly on the gurney, I started to feel slightly better. My breathing had normalized. After a few minutes, the weakness began to pass and I was sure I could get up and go back to the surgery. When I opened my eyes, everything looked normal.

Slowly, I sat up, stretched, and still felt all right. "I'm okay now," I said aloud. I started to get off the gurney, but the doctor laid his hand on my shoulder and shook his head. "Wait."

"I feel fine."

"Let's be sure," he said.

Although I wanted to protest, I knew he was right. I lay down and closed my eyes. I waited, sure I would feel absolutely fine within a few minutes. However, I did not start feeling fine.

"I'm cold," I said. Someone draped a sheet over me and I felt my body relax.

I lost all sense of time, but I do remember that a cardiologist came in and examined me. Nothing seemed abnormal, including my electrocardiogram. He assured me that whatever had happened, it was not my heart. "Everything is normal there," he said.

"That's good to know," I said, reasoning that if it had not been a heart attack, then my condition was not serious.

I thanked him. Then I realized I felt about normal, although tired, so I decided to get up, change, and go home. As I pushed myself to a sitting position, I thought, "I feel as if I've worked a fifteen-hour shift without a break."

"Don't go home, Ben," Dr. Shah, the cardiologist said. "I want to observe you overnight."

I opened my mouth to protest, but he was right. Had the situation been reversed, I would have insisted he stay. I nodded my agreement. Within minutes, a nurse wheeled me into a private room.

---

## *Esther's Reflections . . .*

When my husband collapsed in surgery, I was at church, playing the piano and singing with friends long after the Sabbath services ended. It was as if my soul, unbeknown to me, was storing up nourishment for the difficult journey ahead. When I got home, the phone was ringing. "I'm in the hospital." Ben said on the other end. "Yes, I know," I said. "You're working." "No, I've been admitted," he told me. But I could hear a "smile" in his voice, so I thought he was teasing me. Ben never had been hospitalized before. I only believed him when Dr. Shah called right after to say he was keeping Ben overnight for observation. I rushed to the hospital.

---

When Esther walked into my room, I smiled at her. She returned my smile but asked me a lot of questions.

"What happened? How do you feel? If you feel fine, then why are they keeping you?"

"Just tired," I mumbled. "Just tired, I think."

She sat down next to my bed, held my hand, and we talked a few minutes. I felt too tired to say much. Esther, who is also a nurse, left the room so she could talk to my nurse about my condition.

A vague discomfort came over my entire body. My stomach started to cramp. I relaxed, but the sharp cramping only worsened. Wearily, I got out of bed and went into the bathroom. When I flushed the toilet, I noticed there was blood in my stool. That was odd, because it indicated internal bleeding of some kind. Yet I felt all right, and the blood did not seem important. Or maybe I did not want it to be important. Right then, I was too tired to think of medical indications. I just wanted to get back to the bed and rest.

When Esther returned, I told her, "I had a tarry (clotted blood) stool."

"What did you do with it?" she asked.

"I flushed it."

"You flushed it? Did you tell your nurse?"

"No, it's not important," I said.

"It is important," she said.

Esther was right.

As a medical doctor, I tried to analyze my own condition. I had been trying to convince myself that whatever was keeping me at the hospital for observation could not be anything serious. If so, would I not have known? Would I not have had symptoms before? Pain? Tiredness? Previous weakness? Or anything that would alert me? "This came on too suddenly. It can't be anything serious," I kept saying to myself.

But now one thing nagged at the back of my mind: the blood in my stool. Other than a little cramping, I felt no discomfort or pain. I refused to think about the possibilities of anything being wrong internally because I did not want to get worried about serious—really serious possibilities.

Later, when lying alone in my darkened room, the one terrifying word that I had pushed aside and refused to consider finally reached my consciousness: Cancer.

"My husband has blood in his stool," I heard Esther tell a nurse. "Please make sure the doctor knows."

The nurse reported the blood, and they scheduled a stool test right away for internal bleeding. It was positive.

When the nurse asked me questions, I admitted that yes, in the previous months, I suffered occasionally from indigestion. "Always short-lived and not severe," I added.

Although I did not tell her, I assumed it was something minor, such as hiatal hernia. When indigestion came on, I would drink a lot of water. Sometimes I had a coke or cup of coffee. The discomfort would then go away immediately. Because it went away, I did not allow myself to think about it.

Just before midnight, Esther made sure I was comfortable and had no pain before saying she wanted to go home and get some rest. She had been there for hours. She did not tell me, but that was not the true reason she wanted to leave. Esther had been trained as a nurse. Even before the test results came, she knew I had cancer. She did not

17

nse her true feelings. She reasoned that if she could get
, ...self, to pray, and to find strength from God, she could cope
with whatever happened.

Neither of us said the word to each other, and we did not talk
about my condition. To talk about it would have been too difficult for
either of us that night.

---

### *Esther's Reflections...*

When Ben told me he had blood in his stool, I remembered the bleeding he mentioned that morning inside his mouth,
and the first thing I thought about was cancer. But where? I sat
quietly holding Ben's hand, I thought about the long, intense
suffering of the woman cancer patient I had tended as a nurse
in California. I was afraid, and I did not want to see Ben suffer
like that. I wanted to cry, but I held on until he was ready to
sleep. Then, I went home and jumped on the bed. I screamed
and cried. I prayed and called my parents, brother Sam, sisters
and a friend, Jeanne Melashenko. Then, I cried myself to sleep.

---

As I lay in bed, haunted by the prospect of terminal illness, I
recalled the strange feelings I had while shaving on the morning of my
birthday. Feelings of emptiness, a deep longing, a lack of fulfillment.
For the first time, I admitted that something definitely was missing in
my life, but I had no idea what it was. "Strange to think that way,"
I thought. After all, I was living the American dream. I had a wife,
three fine, grown kids, and a solid medical practice. I had handled my
finances and investments well, and my health had always been good.
Was it really possible that I might have a debilitating and life-threatening illness? Was it too late for me to figure out what was lacking in
my life, and to do something about it?

I regretted not taking better care of myself. Esther was a vegetarian and conscious of healthy living, so my lifestyle had troubled
her. I stayed too busy to worry about such things. Esther had been telling me quietly for years that I was not eating right: "Take time to eat.
Enjoy your meal and chew your food well. Eat more fruits and vegetables. Stay away from coffee and sweets.

"Oh, I know you're right," I would always say, but no changes.

Esther also was more committed spiritually than I was. My parents had raised me as a strict Seventh-day Adventist; I had never left the church or turned from faith in Jesus Christ. I believed in God and I was a church member, but I did not have the kind of commitment and faith that Esther had. God was part of my life but just was not all-important to me. I did not go to church often because of my weekend duties. After all, I reasoned, I served God when I worked on the Sabbath.

In my hospital bed, as I reviewed my thoughts of only four days before, I almost laughed. That morning I had asked, "Okay, God, now what? What do you want me to do with my life?"

Was this the answer God was giving me? To be sick? To face physical problems? Being a patient in a hospital bed was not the kind of answer I had expected—or wanted, especially an answer that included the possibility of having cancer.

Never in my life had there been a time when I did not believe in God's love for me. But on this night, I felt distant, alone and frightened. I desperately wanted to feel God's presence.

Exhausted, I drifted off to sleep.

The next morning, a surgeon I knew well, Dr. Frederick Winegarner, came in to see me. Because he had not examined me, he did not know what was wrong. I did not offer any suggestions—as if my not speaking about my worst fear would make it go away. Even though a deep, inner part of me was certain, I wanted to be mistaken about my self-diagnosis.

"I'm going to insert a scope and see if I can locate the cause of the bleeding," he said.

That was standard procedure so I agreed. He would have to put me under deep sedation and then insert a long tube called an endoscope, down my throat.

When I awakened, Dr. Winegarner was still in the endoscopy room studying the pictures. He later told Esther when he looked down the endoscope into my stomach, there were tears in his eyes.

"What did you find?" I asked. For several seconds, he said nothing but stared at the pictures. His silence confirmed what I already knew.

"Is it cancer?"

He hesitated and then said, sadly, "Yes, I'm sorry, Ben."

"Where?"

"It's in the lower part of your esophagus."

"Oh," I said quietly. Both of us knew the weakness and fainting in the operating room happened because I had been bleeding internally, and the bleeding must have been going on for some time. By then I was ready to hear the diagnosis. But, I was not as ready to hear the location: The esophagus (the passageway of food from the mouth to the stomach).

---

### *Esther's Reflections...*

Early the next morning before he performed the endoscopy on Ben, Dr. Winegarner said he'd see me in 10 minutes. Thirty minutes later, my heart was pumping so fast. I kept wondering, "What's going on?"

I walked into the scope room without even asking permission. Everyone was silent. Ben was facing the window, looking at the pictures taken internally by the scope's tiny camera. I wanted to break the silence by screaming. I touched Ben's head and he turned to me. "Honey, it's positive," he said.

I could not find words to say or tears to shed. Then, I just followed as they wheeled Ben to his room. Ben and I just sat quietly, looking at each other. As the nurses, doctors, and other people came in and out, I sat in a corner and watched. All I heard were words "cancer" and "death" over and over. I decided I had to think positively. I am going to focus on God because God can do miracles.

---

Although esophageal cancer is fairly rare, I knew what to expect. In patients I had seen personally, the surgeon removed the cancer, but in almost all cases it had already spread before it was diagnosed. I never saw anyone with esophageal cancer in our hospital that survived more than a few months.

Right then I lost all interest in living.

Dr. Winegarner pointed to the growth on the pictures which

showed the tumor obstructing a third of the esophageal lumen (opening). Although he tried to encourage me because the tumor was small, we both knew it was growing rapidly. Very rapidly. Within weeks—if left untreated—the pain would become intense and the growth would obstruct the esophagus so that no food could get in. It was only a question of time.

Surgery seemed the only option, but, at best, it would give me a little more time and make my last days less painful. Yes, I thought, surgery will buy me a little time, but that is all.

As they wheeled me back to my room, one part of my mind kept saying, "It's terminal. I'm going to die." Another part of me kept saying, "No, no, no. He's made a mistake. He read the scope pictures wrong."

In my room, and now fully awake, I stared at the ceiling. I knew I should pray, to ask God for help, to plead for mercy, but I did not. "Well, this is it," I thought. "It's been diagnosed as esophageal cancer. I'm going to die."

When Dr. Winegarner returned after getting the biopsy, he sat on the corner of my bed. "They have to remove that lesion, Ben. I'd like to send you to the best hospital in Ohio. I'd like you to have the best surgeon, and then we go from there." In his opinion, those were: The Arthur James Cancer Center at Columbus and Dr. Christopher Ellison, Chief Surgeon of the Surgical Department at the Ohio State University.

"All right," I said, but I knew it did not matter where I went for treatment. The end would be the same. Outwardly, I became a cooperative patient. I had worked beside surgeons in thousands of operations and I knew how hard they tried. I wanted to cooperate, not disappoint them. Inwardly, I kept thinking, "It doesn't matter what they do. Nothing will help."

Although he did not say the words, Dr. Winegarner implied that after surgery, I would have to undergo chemotherapy and radiation, which were the next steps in the normal treatment for any cancer.

As a lifelong Adventist, I had heard of alternative forms of medicine, thought about them, and had quietly dismissed them. What difference did it make what I did? I was going to die anyway.

Dr. Winegarner called Dr. Ellison and asked if he could see me right away. Usually it takes weeks to be scheduled for surgery in

Columbus. He agreed to see me within hours.

The fighting and the waiting began.

After my diagnosis, Esther wanted me to have surgery at Loma Linda University in Southern California, one of the most prestigious hospitals in our denomination and one that has done outstanding work in cancer treatment. She also wanted the presence and support of her family who lives there. I felt torn between going to Columbus and Loma Linda.

The phone rang with get-well wishes and prayers. Friends, doctors, nurses and hospital personnel came to visit me right away. Esther and my children walked in my room and saw them encircling my bed, hugging, encouraging and offering prayers for me. Many tears were shed.

When Esther became aware of the support and affection for me, she said, "Honey, Marion is home for you. You'll get the love and support and care you need here. At Loma Linda, you would be among strangers."

We made our decision I would go to Columbus, fifty miles away. On April 1, one day after my diagnosis, Esther took me to meet Dr. Ellison in Columbus and he examined me. He made several shifts in his schedule and I had to wait only one week. In the mean time, he gave his phone number to call if bleeding started again. More extensive tests were done.

Only when I faced the end of my life did I finally turn to God for help. I prayed with a fervency I had never felt before. "Oh God, please hear me," I began. "I am powerless to face this problem alone."

Despite being a Christian, it was quite a step for me to pull myself together and ask for God's help. Never had I faced a desperate situation before—a situation that was beyond me. All my life I had done everything for myself, worked hard, acquired material things, and believed God then blessed what I did. This time it was different.

To write about this change in my life may make it sound easy or simple. It was neither. I had reached the place where I knew God was my only chance and still I held back from a total surrender of myself. I had failed God so many times and ignored God. However, enough of my childhood teaching and Esther's encouragement made me realize that Jesus Christ would hear me.

I was not sure how to turn to God, so I just opened myself as honestly as I could.

"My Lord, I'm terrified and desperate," I began. "I don't even know the right way to do this, but I'm giving myself to you. Lord, I am sick and I can't help myself. You're in control of my life. What will you have me to do now? What will you allow me to do? Will you allow me to die? Will you allow me to suffer?"

As I poured out my heart to God, I thought of Esther. I had not always been a good husband. Too often I had neglected her. I had stayed so busy in my practice that sometimes I practically left her alone to take care of our children. One time I was even unfaithful to her. Esther never threatened to leave me or made me feel she had ever stopped loving me. After some difficult struggles in the 1980s, I had tried to be a better husband by spending more time with her. I wanted to be even closer to her now.

"Oh, God, please give me time for us to make it up, for me to be the kind of husband Esther deserves," I prayed.

As I prayed, I realized—for the first time in years—how much I loved that woman. When she came into my room, I hugged her. "I love you," I said through tears. "Please forgive me."

As we held each other, our tears mingled. "I love you, too, and I forgive you," she said.

When I heard those words and knew she meant them, I knew I was ready and determined to straighten out my life in the remaining time I had left. I was positive I would die soon—months at the longest—but I wanted those days to be devoted to the woman who had devoted herself so unselfishly to me.

"Before I die, Lord, please help me," I asked. "Help me draw closer to Esther, the kids and to you."

I had no idea how God would answer that prayer. I did not even know for sure if God heard me.

### Esther's Reflections...

At first, I did not want Ben to have surgery, even after discussing the matter with my children. I just wanted to take him away on vacation with them. But because of the internal bleeding, I knew he must have the surgery. Still, I kept saying to myself, "What can anyone do? It is cancer." Then, many of the physicians from both hospitals in Marion (which then were rivals) came to give support. It was amazing! It really did give me hope, especially after Dr. Hering took his time and helped me decide whether to bring Ben to California or remain in Ohio. (Dr. James Hering, Surgeon, helped Ben start his private practice in Marion).

I called more people to pray for Ben. It reminded me of the woman who touched Jesus' garment. Her faith made her well. So, I tried to stay strong for my husband and my children. I kept praying and hoping that he would not give up. I knew we could fight this together.

I begged God for Ben's life. Then I thought many times about my father's comment to me the night before: "God gave Ben to you and He can also take him away from you. Let's put things in God's hands." So I prayed, "If you take him away from me then please give us one more year." But at the same time I was also thinking, "It can't be. I want him to stay alive." Then I thought about what had happened to his esophagus. How can he eat and drink? "Oh," I thought, "I won't mind taking care of him and will keep feeding him through a tube." But my fear was, "What if he gives up?" Oh, I just wanted to rest my mind and not think about anything. I decided to take things a day at a time. There were times that I wanted to really scream and cry out loud. But I did not want him to see my pain.

When Ben was discharged from Marion General Hospital after the endoscopic exam, we spent the next few days acting as if nothing dreadful happened. We tried to work normally. He told me about things that I needed to know...paper work, documents, insurance. But at that time, I did not want to hear any of those things. I just wanted to be with him. We did not say much, except, "I love you," which we said numerous times. I also wanted to rest and sleep, with him beside me.

The week was very busy with phone calls; visitors and relatives arriving; more lab tests; paper work. People came to pray, sing and worship with us in our home. Saturday night before Ben's surgery, our church pastor anointed Ben with oil. All I thought at this time was that Ben would make it, although he would have some difficulties. I was determined to prepare myself to make things easier for him. I thought of bringing him to visit gardens with plenty of beautiful flowers and plants...hiking...bird watching, and walks under the sunlight. I did not want to think about death. I totally removed that word from my thoughts. Instead, I focused on things I would do to help him cope with the post-surgical pain, the intravenous fluids, the tube feedings, getting him out of bed, and giving him a bath. It never crossed my mind that I was being selfish. I just felt I could not give him up.

# Ben's Beginnings

*"Train up a child in the way he should go: and when he is old,
he will not depart from it."*
—Proverbs 22:6 (KJV)

## My Homeland's History

For people to understand my life and me, they need to know some of the history of the Republic of the Philippines. This is an overview of the history in which I grew up.

Spain ruled the Philippine Islands from the time Magellan landed in 1521 until American's Admiral Dewey defeated the Spanish forces in 1898. The series of islands remained under the control of the United States. In 1934, the country was granted its commonwealth status to end on July 4, 1946. In 1935, Manuel Quezon was elected the first president for a six-year term.

On the morning of December 8, 1941 (Manila time), when the Japanese bombed Pearl Harbor, they also invaded the Philippines. After one month of resistance, Manila fell, and shortly afterward, the American military forces surrendered at Bataan and then at Corregidor. When Gen. Douglas MacArthur and his troops left, the General stood in the waters, turned back, and cried out, "I shall return."

His words became a symbol of unity, and the people of the Philippines rallied behind that promise.

Many Americans, unable to flee, were imprisoned; most

of them died before the war ended. President Quezon transferred his government to Washington. Filipinos left on the island had to care for themselves, and some chose to collaborate with the Japanese. Others carried on guerrilla war against the enemy from the jungles and the mountains. In 1943, the tide of war turned and Filipinos began to dream of freedom once again.

After much bombing and naval activity, under Gen. MacArthur, US forces landed at Leyte on October 20, 1944. On February 1945, US forces entered Manila. For three weeks, the Japanese-occupied section of Intramuros was the scene of fires and fighting and was sacked by the Japanese in a ruthless orgy of rape, destruction, and bloodshed. Fierce fighting filled the islands, with thousands of deaths on both sides, before the Japanese surrendered.

President Quezon died in 1944, before the liberation of his country. MacArthur and then-president Osmena administered commonwealth affairs during the difficult transition between war and peace. To the Filipino people, MacArthur was hailed as their liberator. The United States officially granted independence to the Republic of the Philippines on July 4, 1946.

I was born March 26, 1945, in Narvacan, Ilocus Sur, a town in Northern Luzon, during the closing days of World War II. Before the war, my father, Benjamin C. Sanidad, Sr., was a high school teacher in a school operated by the Seventh-day Adventist church. He had always been a faithful Adventist. After the Japanese invaded, he joined the Philippine guerillas and was commissioned in the army as a Sergeant. Because the Japanese accused him of helping their enemy, they imprisoned him.

The Japanese had come into the country saying they had no quarrel with the Filipinos. They claimed they only wanted to chase out the Americans the way the Americans had chased out the Spaniards. Once they assumed power, however, the Japanese treated the people badly: robbing, beating, raping, mistreating, and killing them.

Conditions in the country continued to worsen as the new rulers bore down heavily on the people. For the next three years, many Filipinos carried on a battle of wits with their conquerors—lying, cheating, and stealing—whatever was necessary to preserve their lives.

I was born in an evacuation center in the mountains. Because there were no houses, my mother gave birth to me in a thatched hut. Dad still served with the military and was away. Mom sent word of my birth, but he did not get to come home for another week.

My parents named me Benjamin, after my father. They nicknamed me after General MacArthur, who had already become a symbol of freedom to the Filipino people. From my first days, mom began to call me "Arthur." Even now, more than 50 years later, she still calls me by that name.

The war in the Pacific ended in August 1945. The people were poor and impoverished; the land had been gutted and devastated. American aid helped our country immensely in a recovery program that continued until 1954.

As soon as the war was over, the three of us moved to Artacho, Sison, Pangasinan in Luzon, which is north of Manila. Dad received an appointment to teach in the same Adventist school where he had taught before the war.

The school at Northern Luzon Academy became home to me and to my three sisters and a brother born after me. We spent all our growing-up years in this sprawling compound situated in a valley surrounded by mountain ranges and a river close by. Then we bought land just outside the southern part of the campus. Many different kinds of fruit trees were growing in this prime land: coconuts, caimitos, sineguelas, mangos, guayabanos, guavas, chicos, carmay, pomelos and others. The whole year round, we climbed these trees and harvested varieties of fruits which we enjoyed eating.

Although I remember few details of my childhood, it was a happy time. Mom taught me to read and to enjoy both words and pictures. I learned to count and absorbed the beginning concepts of the meaning of numbers before I entered school.

When I turned five, mom enrolled me in the school's kindergarten program. Like most five-year-old children, I did not want to stay inside a classroom all day, but mom insisted, so I went into the room, absolutely sure I would hate it. By the end of the first day, however, I began to enjoy being with other children and made a number of friends. Soon I looked forward to going to school each day.

The following year, mom enrolled me in grade one. After the first day, the teacher objected. "He does not belong in grade one," she said to my mother. "He already knows everything I am teaching." She had observed me the previous year and realized even then that I was advanced.

Her remarks about my development caused a bit of discussion, as my parents reminded me later. At first they were not sure what to do. Finally, instead of entering grade one, I went into grade two at age six. That made me at least a year younger than my classmates, but I have no sense of having suffered from that fact. Part of the reason may have been that we lived in the school compound, and in many ways we were like an extended family. So far as I know, everyone accepted me as I was.

The school system in the Philippines differs from that of the United States. We went to elementary school for grades one through six. After that, we attended high school for four more years, making it a total of ten years of formal education. By the time I was eleven years old, I graduated from elementary school, and that same year I entered high school. They told me I was a "driven" student, and I probably was. I wanted to please my parents, and I wanted to please myself too. Perhaps on some level I worked harder to prove myself because I was younger, although I was not aware of feeling that way.

I do know that I figured out something quite early: The harder I worked, the more I pleased my parents as well as my teachers. I saw the rewards of being a good student. When I did well, the teachers and my parents complimented me.

All five of us children felt close to each other, and were taught to help our parents in doing chores at home. My dad taught my brother and me to plant fruit trees, to garden, and how to raise chickens and goats. The girls helped my mom and divided their duties at home between cleaning the house, hand-washing clothes, and helping to prepare food for the family.

From time to time in our family, we talked about my future. Dad thought I would do well as a lawyer, but mom really wanted me to be a doctor. During my childhood, I listened when they talked to me about what I would eventually do for a career, but being young, I did not think much about the future.

For almost a decade after World War II, the US military seemed everywhere in our country. I especially remember hearing planes coming in and going out all hours of the day or night. Those planes fascinated me and I tried to figure out how it would feel to fly an airplane high above the clouds. I learned to make toy airplanes. I thought being a pilot was the most wonderful job I could ever have. (*It was not until I was in my forties that I finally found out when I learned to fly a plane.*)

Another influence in my life was my Uncle David, mom's brother. He was a general surgeon who left the Philippines and went to the United States right after the end of World War II. He became a respected and well-known practitioner in the San Francisco area in California.

It seemed to me as a child that mom constantly talked about him and she was proud of what he had done with his life. I am sure she actually did not, but it was frequently enough that I thought about him often. Uncle David became a hero to me. Mom often told me about his work and the wonderful things he was doing. After Uncle David had immigrated to the United States, he sent us many American-made goods—very expensive and difficult to get in those days.

More than that, I remember the pictures he sent. As my eyes scanned each postcard, I realized what a beautiful land America was. He wrote about everyone having telephones in their homes and about cars that went extremely fast. I could hardly believe it when he wrote that everyone in the United States had electricity, even in the most remote places. So many places in our country did not have any of those things, so I knew it must be a wonderful place. Even as a young boy, I wanted to be like Uncle David and see all those things and places.

From that desire, it seemed obvious to me as early as eight years of age that if I became a doctor, I could go to America like my uncle, buy a fast car, ride on a train, and have a telephone in my home.

"I want to be a doctor," I told my parents one day. I did not tell them that wanting things such as cars and telephones was what made me choose medicine. Many years later I would be reminded that my whole life had built itself around acquiring the things I had dreamed of when I was eight years old.

"That is a wonderful choice," my mother said.

Dad never opposed my choice of medicine, as I remember, because he was not like that. He wanted the best career possible for me.

So it was settled: Ben would become a doctor.

Another thing that fascinated me was politics. Relatives on both sides of my family had already gone into politics, one of whom was a Senator. On mom's side, we were related to Ferdinand Marcos. I watched the rise of Marcos, who started out in the Philippine Congress and was a highly respected Senator for many years. Eventually, of course, he became the President.

For me, politics meant being in front, winning, and especially being in a position to make decisions that affected others, such as classmates.

"I am going to be at the top of my class," I vowed to myself. It was not something I told anyone, but I decided that is what I would do. Usually, the students who are at the top of the class are leaders and get a lot of recognition in school activities. That is what politics was—being a leader—and I liked to be a leader.

At age eleven, I entered high school. Just as in elementary school, I felt strongly motivated to study hard. I decided that I would be at the top of my class in every subject. Now, years later as I reflect on those days, I am thankful that God gave me opportunities to excel as a school leader as well as the intellectual capacity to do quality work that earned me the highest grades.

Just as I had planned, I worked hard and made some of the highest grades in the school. I maintained that record all through the four years of high school.

Despite my academic achievements, all during high school my interest in politics remained. Again, that may have been because of family involvement, but the subject always fascinated me. From my earliest grades in school, I ran for various school offices—usually class president—but whatever it was, I always won. In high school, the other students elected me class president each of my four years. Although I loved politics and the activities that it involved me in, I never neglected my studies.

I loved the environment of sharing ideas and challenging people to make decisions. Several times in school, I seriously thought about entering the political life. With the right encouragement, I might have gone that way. Instead, I moved forward in my choice of a medical career.

\* \* \*

All through childhood, I lived in a conservative Christian home. My ten years of schooling were all in Adventists-operated schools where Bible and health were part of our everyday studies. Not only were my parents Christians and faithful to the church, but also they tried to instill in each of us children a love for God. Even today, I still remember the worship together in the mornings and again in the evenings. I never questioned whether to do it or its value. We just worshiped because it was part of our daily routine. I did not know then that all Christians did not have daily worship, or even that not all Adventists did. I assumed that the way we lived was exactly like all the others did.

At no time did I ever openly rebel against what my parents taught me. In some ways, it might have been better if I had rebelled—it might have made me face myself earlier. No, I lived a good moral life and behaved like everyone else I knew. Because I acted properly, no one questioned my relationship to Jesus Christ. Inwardly, however, I never really surrendered my life to God.

Despite their attempts to teach me, I was not really a Christian, in the sense of being faithful to obey God's commands. Family worship and church activities were simply things I did, but they did not engage my heart, only my actions.

At times I prayed—each of the Sanidad children learned to do that before we could read. I learned to say things such as, "Lord, give me strength..." "Dear Father, give me the knowledge to know how to..." "Loving God, forgive me for..." I knew all the right words along with the proper way to behave.

The reality, however, was that I believed I could do just about anything by myself. I did not particularly need God's help, although I would never have said so. All through school I had proven to myself that I could do anything I needed or wanted if I worked at it hard enough.

My parents continued to faithfully plant the right seeds. It took a long time—fifty years—for those seeds to mature and bear fruit. That does not mean I dropped out of church, because I did not. I did everything the other kids did. Later, after I started my medical practice, my church attendance became infrequent, but I used my work as my excuse. No one ever challenged me or asked if I was putting my career ahead of God.

Like the other young people my age, I received water baptism in our church. It happened during my first year of high school. As was the custom, we had our regular classes during the day, but for six nights, we had evangelistic services, which they called a "Week of Prayer." A Filipino minister from Hawaii, preached every night. As he stood before us, his eyes filled with fire and his voice with passion, he focused his messages on us students.

As I remember, it was not a matter of choosing to go or not to go. The faculty, parents, and all the students assumed everyone would attend, even though I don't think anyone ever said we had to. It was simply understood that we would be there.

During Pastor Basconcillo's last message, he made a strong point that we had to believe in Jesus Christ or we were not Christians, even if we were good students in the school. He paused and then asked, "How many of you believe in Jesus Christ as the Lord and your Savior?"

Every kid's hand shot up. Mine went right there with the others.

"But that is not enough," he said. "Once you have turned to Jesus Christ, you must take the first step of obedience." He explained the meaning and the importance of baptism. Then he paused and his eyes moved around the large chapel. "How many of you would like to be baptized?" he asked.

I raised my hand. So did others, maybe a total of twenty of us. Most of the older kids had been baptized already.

Apparently our teachers thought we were ready for baptism. After all, each of us came from a Christian home and our parents had sent us to a Christian school. The next day, Saturday afternoon, the pastor held a ceremony at a nearby river because Adventists practice immersion. After all of us had been baptized, Pastor Basconcillo and the teachers welcomed us into the church as true believers.

I had no questions about what I was doing. It seemed like the right thing to do. From childhood, I had known that one day my parents expected me to do certain things such as profess faith in Jesus Christ, be immersed, and join the church. It was not a significant experience for me, as I am sure it was for some. Perhaps if it had happened in college, or when I was older, I might have thought more about it. Or at least I might have hesitated before I agreed to being baptized and joining the church.

\* \* \*

Money was not plentiful in those days, but our family lived as well as any of the others we knew. Because my father was a teacher—a "worker" as they called him—he received a 40 percent discount on the tuition for each of his children.

Dad's father, who was a farmer, provided a lot of the food we ate. He also promised to help me with my college tuition after graduation from high school. Then my training would begin and I would be ready to face the world and build my career.

I did not know it, but the influence of God was beginning to lessen in my life.

## MY PARENTS

*(My aunt, Consuelo Roda Jackson, wrote the following account of how my parents married. My mom's name is also ESTHER and my dad's name is also BENJAMIN)*

Nana (aunt) Maming awakened Esther early on the morning of April 10, 1944. She hated to tell her niece the terrible news. When they first learned, she and her husband had agreed not to tell Esther until the next morning.

Months earlier, the Japanese had declared peace and mandated schools to re-open. Although only 18, Esther de la Cruz

Roda was one of the young women chosen to teach. When the summer break came, she went to Artacho, Pangasinan, a town north of Manila to attend a workshop for Adventist teachers. She stayed in the home of her Uncle Tony.

"We should have awakened you last night," her aunt said, "but you needed all the sleep you could get, so we decided to wait." Forcing herself not to cry, she laid her hands on Esther's shoulder. "Anak (child), Japanese soldiers came last night."

Esther stared, waiting for the rest of the message.

"They took Ben away."

"Oh, no—" she said. Esther's world had suddenly turned dark. A dizziness came over her and she leaned against the wall for support.

"Where is he now?" she asked.

"We do not know." Nana Maming hugged her niece. "Anak, we think they have taken him to the garrison in Urdaneta."(*Another town north of Artacho*).

Ben had come to see Esther—the first meeting after he left their evacuation camp. He had told her about a harrowing experience he had shared with Esther's older brother David and Ben's Uncle Rodolfo. Adventurous by nature, and curious to see the aftermath of the battle, the three decided to return to Northern Luzon Academy in Artacho (*where Ben was a teacher*). Within hours of their return, Japanese soldiers arrested all three at bayonet point. Unless proven otherwise, the Japanese regarded all Filipinos as enemies.

All three tried to explain they were not enemies, but the soldiers refused to listen. In their searching the men, they found a bundle of papers that Ben was carrying. They demanded to know what they were.

"My letters—letters I wrote to my sweetheart," Ben said. "I found them in the rubble of her home, which had been burned to the ground."

The letters convinced them that Ben was indeed a teacher. On the strength of those letters, the soldiers released them. They knew the soldiers could just have easily taken them prisoners.

That same evening, Ben had proposed to Esther.

"I'm only eighteen years old," she reminded Ben, who was seven years older. "I'd like to finish my education before getting married."

When they said good night, Ben's disappointment was obvious. Esther loved him, but she felt she was just too young.

As she listened to her uncle and aunt, Esther realized Ben's life was in danger. Being interred by the Japanese meant he might not get out. He could die there.

"Lord, show us what to do for Ben," she prayed. Just then, into her mind flashed the story of Queen Esther, whose people, already captives of the Persians, now faced death. A newly enacted law gave Persians the right to kill Jews. Queen Esther knew that the only way to save them was for her to risk her own life to reveal to the king that she was a Jew and plead for mercy.

Queen Esther's Uncle Mordecai had challenged her by saying, "Who knows but that you have come to the royal position for such a time as this?" She had decided to do that and said, "If I perish, I perish."

Like the ancient queen, Esther knew what she was to do. "I'll go to the garrison," she said.

They had one chance—for her to plead for them to release Ben so they could marry. Even though she had not felt ready, Ben's life was more important than her plans.

The school and Mission leaders agreed with her. Professor Tomas Pilar, one of Ben's former teachers, offered to go with her. They hired a *kalesa* (a horse-drawn cart), the only transportation available.

On their way to Urdaneta, they came upon an army truck parked in the hot sun and away from any shade. Esther gasped as she looked at the sight. In the back of the truck she spotted Ben and others, but her attention was only on him. They had obviously beaten him—he had bruises all over his face and his eyes were almost shut. They had tied his hands.

She walked near the truck, and without stopping or speaking to Ben, she said to one of the soldiers, "We are going to the garrison." She assumed Ben heard her words and recognized her voice.

When they arrived at the garrison, Esther saw the army truck had taken another road and had already arrived there. It was again parked in the sun. Ben and the others were still there and still tied. Again she walked up to the truck without turning to address Ben. She said to one of the soldiers, "We wish to see the *Kempetai* (commanding officer)."

The guard pointed the way to the commander's office. As she and Professor Pilar walked forward, she prayed silently. "Thank you for leading us thus far. You hold the universe in your hands, Lord, and to you, nothing is impossible. Enable us to speak only the right words. Bless this officer, too, Lord. Touch his heart."

The commander made them wait for three days. They sat all day outside his office. Finally, he called them into his office. Esther curtsied to the officer, and then explained why she had come.

"He is not from this area. He came only to see me," she said.

Professor Pilar told the officer that Ben, who was a teacher, had come into the area to marry Esther, his sweetheart, who was also a teacher.

In fluent English, the commander asked Esther many questions, such as, "So you are a teacher, are you? When did you arrive for the workshop? When did your boyfriend arrive?" He continued for a long time and then finally asked, "When are you getting married?"

When Esther hesitated, Professor Pilar, who was an ordained minister, said, "As soon as Ben is released, I will perform their wedding."

"Is that so?" he asked Esther.

She nodded.

"All right, teacher, I want you to be happy. You go home now. Tomorrow,

we will free your sweetheart so you can get married."

They thanked the commander respectfully and left.

Before they left for the garrison, Professor Pilar had sent word to Esther's parents, advising them to come immediately. He believed that if Esther agreed to the marriage, it would save Ben's life. He wanted Esther's parents there in case the officer himself or one of his representatives decided to come.

True to his word, the Japanese officer released Ben.

"How did you get those bruises?" was one of Esther's first questions when she saw her future husband.

"The day after I came to see you the Japanese came where I was staying. They demanded that I take them to my followers," he said.

"They did not believe me when I told them I was not a guerilla and that I had no followers." Ben kept denying their charges and they insisted he was lying.

"They kicked me, slapped me, and then tied my hands behind me. They pushed me to the ground on my back. 'Drink,' one of them ordered as he poured water into my mouth. This went on a long time and they kept telling me to drink. When my abdomen became distended, and I could drink no more, the soldier kicked me repeatedly in the abdomen. Water gushed out my mouth. Again they forced me to drink more water and then they kicked my abdomen. They did this many times, saying they would keep repeating the treatment until I confessed."

"Unable to extract what they wanted, they took me to the long bridge and held me over the side. I saw rocks below and knew the fall would kill me. I pleaded with them, but they would not believe me. They picked me up and flung me over the bridge. 'God, save me!' I cried.

"My right foot caught on the guardrail. I hung there, pleading for mercy.

"The Lord touched the soldiers' hearts and they helped me get up. As soon as I was on the ground again, they went back to the same kind of torture of kicking, pushing, slapping, and even spitting on my face. One of them grabbed a stick and started jabbing at my eyes. The Lord continued to protect me because the stick never hit my eyes. Then they ordered me to the back of the army truck. With my hands still tied, I got into the truck. I had no idea where they were taking me; I only knew the treatment they gave me was usually the prelude to execution."

He learned later that someone reported to the Japanese officers that he was a guerilla leader who came into the area to organize nationals to oppose the Japanese.

Ben paused and thought about his ordeal before he added, "When I heard your voice, I thought I was dreaming, but I realized I was not. Just to see you brought a great sense of comfort. Now you are truly my Queen Esther. With you, my love, I will serve Him all my life."

On April 16, 1944, the third day after his release, Ben and Esther had a simple, late-afternoon wedding ceremony.

They had released Ben and for now he was safe. But what would happen the next time? Ben, Esther, and all the Christian leaders felt there was only one answer—Ben and Esther must hide in the mountains and work with the guerillas until General MacArthur's forces returned.

As they had planned, the couple sneaked up into the mountains and joined with others who opposed Japan. They stayed there for the next three years.

When the Americans returned in late 1944, my father and many others in the mountains worked with the Allies in a joint Philippine-American program.

# College and Looking Beyond

*"God demands vigorous and earnest intellectual effort, and with
every determined effort, your powers will strengthen.
Put your highest powers into your effort. You are learning. Endeavor
to go to the bottom of everything you set your hand to. Never aim
lower than to become competent in the matters which occupy you."*
—MS 24 1887

At age fifteen, I graduated from high school. Without any question or discussion in our family, the next thing meant I started college.

College would be a big step for me. For one thing, I had never lived away from home and going to college meant moving to Manila. I would attend Philippine Union College, the closest college operated by the Seventh-day Adventists. The school was only 200 kilometers away (*about 160 miles*), but for a boy of my age, it seemed like the school was far and hundreds of miles away.

Our denomination had two colleges, but I do not recall that we even discussed my going anywhere else. Everyone seemed to assume that those who graduated from Northern Luzon Academy and went on to college would enroll at Philippine Union College.

My parents would never have agreed for me to attend a public college because, like most Seventh Day Adventists, they believed that only in our own school system could their children receive balanced education for our "social, physical, mental and spiritual powers."

My new life had begun.

\* \* \*

When still a child, I had decided to become a doctor because of my Uncle Dave's influence. Along with that decision, I knew I wanted to get my medical education in the United States.

Other than a few thoughts about the possibility of entering politics, I knew that medicine was where I wanted to direct my career. The desire to be a doctor never left me.

My dad took me to Manila by bus and stayed with me until I was enrolled at the Philippine Union College. I felt a little hesitancy during enrollment—jitters over being in a new environment, meeting new teachers, and not knowing many of my classmates. Even though I was a little anxious, I did not have any real fear or worry, because I knew I would do well in college if I kept on studying the way I had in high school.

I liked college and look back at it as one of the most exciting periods of my life. I thoroughly enjoyed involving myself in a number of extra-curricular activities. All the time, however, I kept my eyes focused on getting the top grades and earning my degree. That was my one goal.

During my second year, I wanted to join the staff of the "College Voice"—the school's monthly newspaper.

"Sorry, but I can't use you," the editor, who was a senior, said to me.

"Why not?"

"You don't have any experience. You've never done any writing or reporting."

I wanted to be on the staff. His turning me down only made me more determined. So I looked right into his eyes and asked, "What does it take to be a member of your editorial staff?"

"Well, you have to have experience as a reporter." From the way he smiled I knew he had not taken me seriously. "First thing, you have to go through a journalism class."

"That's what I'll do, and then I'll be back." Although I said the words to him, I was making a promise to myself.

It was too late to do anything on the "College Voice" or change classes during my second year, but when I signed up for third-year classes, I enrolled in journalism. I loved the class and I learned a great deal about writing and reporting.

When I entered my fourth year of college, I still had my eyes on the "College Voice." Instead of starting at the bottom, I ran for the job of editor, a position voted on by the entire student body. To get that position, I worked hard, ran it like a political campaign and had a lot of fun introducing myself and asking people to vote for me.

I won the election and became the editor for two terms. As I soon learned, the job was more than editing. In my newly won position, I had to appoint reporters, and the job description allowed me to choose my own staff. Because I had enrolled in the journalism classes with an assumption that I would become the editor of the "The College Voice" before I graduated, I had looked around and began privately selecting those I wanted to work with me.

As I planned ahead and made note of those who would do good work on the staff, I realized there were a number of groups on campus. They were distinct factions and organizations with totally different interests and had little in common with other groups. I kept my eyes open for those with ability and leadership within the various organizations who might be willing to help me staff the paper when I became editor. Naturally, I never said a word to any of them.

One person that caught my attention was Cynthia. I liked her because she was smart, intelligent, and a leader in her group. She had a girlfriend named Esther Hernando. When I asked them to be on the staff, to my delight, both accepted.

Besides seeing Cynthia as someone to work on the paper, she became what I called a kind-of a girlfriend.

* * *

In those days at Philippine Union College, we were not allowed to date. We could walk together—as long as we did not hold hands. We had to be careful that we did not become exclusive and spend most of our free time with each other. Cynthia and I did attend college events and other programs, as well as church activities. She was nice to be with, but we never did anything that I would call formal dating.

We did a common boy-girl thing that everyone called marching. That means, we would meet in the campus auditorium on Saturday nights where we would choose our partners. Then we would march to the tune of music—a type of group marching.

At the time, I paid little attention to Esther, although I found her bright, likable, very warm and friendly. We talked casually from time to time, but always in groups. As I learned, she paid part of her college tuition by being a dormitory monitor. Among other things, she had to stay in the parlor whenever boys went over to the girls' dorm. During the dorm's visiting hours, we boys would go over to visit girls, either singly or in small groups. We would talk or walk about the campus but again no formal dating.

One time several other boys and I visited the girls' dorm. Esther sent someone to get the girls. While we waited, Esther and I began to talk. So far as I can remember, it was the first time we had ever talked alone, just the two of us.

To my surprise, she was warmer and funnier than I had suspected. Soon we were teasing each other and laughing. Esther has a wonderful sense of humor and a delightful laugh. During that time— ten minutes at most—we had such a fun time I lost myself and really forgot about Cynthia.

Then I said something—I had not planned to say it and it just popped out—and I have never understood what made me say those words.

"You will not be one of the bride's maids, but you will be the bride," I commented.

I said this in answer to Esther's joking remarks, "I will be one of the bride's maids when you and Cynthia get married."

Esther smiled and I do not recall anything more that we said. But it was the reaction that mattered. To me, it was an attempt at humor; to Esther, it was a serious statement that I wanted to marry her. Neither of us said anything more at the time.

\* \* \*

In college, I wanted to complete my education with top grades so I would be able to enter medical school and go to the United States for further medical training.

In those days, the medical education was not nearly as good in the Philippines as it was in the United States. I assumed I would be a surgeon and, therefore, I wanted the best training available. As everyone knew, as soon as we said, "best training available," we meant going to the United States.

43

Even when I was still a child, I learned it would not be easy to get into the American schools. I often heard talk about others going and it became obvious that the competition was stiff. Knowing that fact pushed me to work extremely hard all the way through school. I reasoned that if I stayed at the academic head of my class, it would open American doors for me.

My commitment and hard work paid off, and I graduated from Philippine Union College with a Bachelor of Science with a major in General Science, a course preparatory for medicine, in 1965, a few weeks after my twentieth birthday.

I started medical school in the summer of 1965 at Manila Central University in Caloocan City, just outside the capital city of Manila. Although not operated by the SDA church, the school catered to Seventh-day Adventist students by allowing them to have classes Sunday through Friday so we could observe the Sabbath on Saturday. Of course, we had to pay for that concession. Teachers received extra money and, because of the extra income, they enjoyed teaching us. However, I chose Manila Central University mainly because three of my doctor uncles were alumni of that school.

Because my dad worked in the denomination at that time as Dean of the boy's dormitory at Philippine Union College, the pay was low, but my parents never complained. My mom was a full-time home keeper and my dad's income strained his paying for my tuition as well as those who followed me. Fortunately for me, my dad's service with the Philippine military forces in World War II provided an educational benefit. The Philippine government provided grants, much like the GI education bill for Americans who served during the war. He had the choice of using it himself or saving it for one of his children. He sacrificed and saved it for me, and he told me about that when I was still in elementary school.

The grant provided a large part of my tuition, so I did not want to disappoint him. That provided the extra incentive to make good grades—which I did.

I finished my four-year medical education in 1969.

By 1965, I had put Philippine Union College behind me. That meant I lost track of Cynthia and Esther and most of the other students.

I applied for my internship and was accepted at The Manila Sanitarium and Hospital, a Seventh-day Adventist institution, and one of the best—if not the best in the Philippines.

I made several applications, one of which was to Clarkfield US Air Force Base, the American hospital in Pampanga. Everybody wanted to go to the United States for training, and going through the American Air Force would be the easiest way to get that training.

Even though I applied, I had a sense—a feeling in my heart is the best way I know to explain it—that even though I would eventually go to the United States, now it was not the right time. When they did not accept me at Clark, I felt no serious disappointment. My time will come, I told myself.

At Manila Sanitarium, as in most medical training facilities, students take rotating internships, that is, they have the opportunity to spend a few months in various forms of medical specialization. In the United States, students who knew the field they wanted to specialize in, could go immediately into training in their area. As required in the Philippines I went through a rotating internship and truly enjoyed every program and gave it my best.

Another incentive to work hard was that at the end of each internship program, the teachers vote for the best intern of the year. My efforts paid off. At the end of the year, they voted me "The Best Intern of The Year," one of the most exciting honors I received.

Life was good for me and I moved along in my career plans as I had expected. I did not think much about God, although I continued to go to church every Sabbath. I felt I obeyed most of the rules and observed them and I felt no different from any other members of the church

In looking back, I know that because I was able, capable, and someone who did well in whatever he tried, I had begun to feel little need for God.

It would be a long time before I realized how needy I really was.

By 1970, by the time I turned twenty-five, I had finished my four years of medical school and my internship. Next came the residency.

# To the USA . . . At Last!

*"Study to show thyself approved unto God; a workman that needeth not to be ashamed, rightly dividing the word of truth."*
—2 Timothy 2:15 (KJV)

While I was still an intern, I applied for training to schools all over the United States—places such as California, New York, Pennsylvania, and Texas. None of them rejected me, but none accepted me either. The sheer volume of applications alone makes it difficult for foreign students to get admitted.

I thought that by applying early, it would give me an advantage. Some schools wrote nice letters and explained that they received so many applications, it was difficult to make decisions and they had only so few slots open.

Many of the institutions did not even reply. I did not quit sending applications, because I never wanted to give up hope.

Among the places I had already applied to was CVS—Cagayan Valley Sanitarium and Hospital—located about a hundred miles northeast from Manila.

If I could not go to the United States, I wanted to be trained at the Manila Sanitarium and Hospital in their four-year surgery residency.

My chances were not good, they offered only one position.

They turned me down, which was quite a blow for my ego and was a stunning disappointment. After all, I had worked hard to hold grades at the top of my class and had the highest recommendations for the post. I also realized, as I had all along, that politics are often overriding factors. I had made good connections, but apparently not quite good enough.

Immediately, I sent new applications to a number of the top medical training institutions in the United States.

While I waited for a reply, a nurse friend called and told me about a conversation between Dr. Celedonio Fernando, who was the director of the hospital at CVS and Dr. Oseas Pilar who headed up the training program. Apparently, Dr. Fernando asked, "Who is your best qualified student?" He, also, explained that he wanted a resident to work with him. "I'd like it to be the best person you have."

"Ben Sanidad," Dr. Pilar answered without hesitating. "He has the highest recommendation of all the staff."

Hours later, Dr. Fernando came to see me. "I'm here to invite you to join me as a resident in Surgery. Would you like to come?"

"I would be honored," I said and meant it. "I can't think of any one I would rather train under."

Dr. Fernando had a reputation as one of the top surgeons in our denomination and in the Philippines. He later became one of the private physicians of the former Philippine President, Ferdinand Marcos.

It was not the hospital I would have chosen, but I ended up with the best man to study under.

In early July of 1970, I packed my things and went to the hospital and started my training program. Almost as soon as I started my training under Dr. Fernando, I realized what a gifted man he was. He deserved his outstanding reputation.

* * *

I had had no contact with Esther after she left for Los Angeles in 1966. If it had not been for other circumstances—and the will of God—she might have been out of my life forever.

Our reconnecting came about in an interesting way. In 1968, when I was a third-year medical student, my brother, Orlando, went to Maryland for a work-study program as a medical technologist. On his way, he stopped over in California to visit Marilyn, his former girl-friend.

Orlando wrote me that Marilyn's roommate was Esther. After

47

that, I began to think a lot more about Esther. I still remembered her well in spite of the four years since we had seen each other. I had always liked her and enjoyed her wonderful sense of humor and pleasant disposition. I decided to write her.

I am not sure of my motives. Maybe it began from loneliness. Money was scarce and I never had enough to take girls out on dates. With my dedication to studies, I did not have time to spend with girlfriends, but I did have time to write a few letters.

I wrote to Marilyn, asking her several questions about Esther. "Is she going with anyone? Does she have a boyfriend? Do you think she would like to hear from me?"

Every afternoon I hurried to check the mail, and the days stretched out. I think it was about 10 days before I received Marilyn's reply. The letter told me exactly the news I had hoped for: "Esther is not going with anyone and has no boyfriend. Yes, I think she would like to hear from you."

In the letter, she wrote about her friendship with Esther, who would soon be taking her board examinations as a Registered Nurse. My heart leaped at one sentence: "I think Esther is lonely and misses the Philippines."

So Esther, too, was lonely.

The more I thought about Esther, the more I really wanted to see her. I already had a desire to go to the U.S., and thinking of Esther made that desire even stronger. If I get there, I thought, I can see Esther.

We began to write back and forth. Most of the time, the same day I received a letter from her, I wrote one back. I liked her letters very much and realized she had matured and become a young woman of great feeling and depth.

Through her letters, I felt as if I knew her and she knew me. I was twenty-five years old, and for the first time, I began to think of marrying her.

Often, as I answered her letters, I asked myself why I had not talked to her more and done things with her when I was in college. But, of course, in those days I had been so focused on getting top grades that relationships were not high on my list of priorities.

To my surprise, I realized that my focus had changed. Despite being involved with Dr. Fernando in an intensive program, I began to think a lot about girls, and especially Esther.

My parents still lived by the old tradition that marriages are family affairs. Parental approval was extremely important. My heart may have been indifferent to God, but I had not rebelled against my family and upbringing. I knew, and I think Esther did as well, that nothing could develop between us without getting both sets of parents to consent.

On a visit home, I talked to mom and dad about my future and where I saw my life going. Then I decided it was time to talk to them about Esther.

"Esther is a good girl," dad said. "Yes, she would be a good choice."

My mom also approved. So it was settled, and now I could talk to Esther's parents and to her.

Perhaps this sounds strange to people outside our culture, but that is how we did things in those days. By then, I was old enough to know that Esther was exactly the kind of woman I wanted to marry. She would be a good wife.

Taking the next step in our tradition, I went to visit her mother. "I would like your permission to correspond with Esther," I said. Although I was already writing to her, I wanted to make it official. After we had spoken a few minutes, I said the words that I had come to declare, "And if God wills, this may lead to marriage."

Her mother, a very straightforward woman, looked directly into my eyes before she said, "Well, we'll pray about it." She did, however, give me permission to write.

Then came the next step, and in some ways the hardest. I am sure it is always hard for a young man to talk to any girl's father. Despite my anxieties, I knew I had to do it.

After I told him my intentions, he treated me kindly. He listened to everything I said and even asked a few questions. Then he said, "Let's pray together." He prayed for me, for Esther, and for any possible union. He did not say so in actual words, but I knew I had also received his permission to correspond with her and to consider talking to her about marriage in the future.

Yes, they approved of our relationship and me. Despite my natural anxieties, I could not think why they would not approve. After all,

I was an Adventist; my father, whom they knew, was a minister and teacher in our schools; I showed promise as a future doctor and could adequately provide for her.

* * *

The letters between Esther and me continued throughout the rest of my third year at Manila Central University and into my fourth. When we began our correspondence, I bought one ream of onionskin paper. Everything went to the U.S. by airmail and the price was based on weight. By using onionskin, I could write three or four pages and send it for what one ordinary sheet of bond paper would cost.

In those days, I had to watch finances carefully. Just the simple act of writing letters regularly to Esther put a drain on my carefully budgeted money. Most of the time I managed with the allowance I received from my parents. But whenever any extra expenses came up, I had no savings or resources to turn to. Many times I ran out of money. I could not ask my parents for more and I absolutely would not try to borrow.

So I did what many other students did to gain a few dollars. From time to time, I went over to the hospital and sold my blood for about two dollars a pint.

Selling my blood every three or four months provided me with money for a few extra things, such as being able to buy the onionskin paper. Occasionally, I sent Esther a few gifts from home. I did not know it then, of course, but Esther saved every letter I wrote her. When we eventually met in the United States, she showed me three bound volumes of my letters. She still has them.

In the exchange of letters, we opened our hearts to each other. I could say things on paper that I probably could not have said if we had been together in person. I felt she understood me and cared. No matter what I wrote, I knew she understood.

At one point in our writing to each other, as a joke and without my knowledge, Orlando wrote a note on the envelope, a gift package (for her graduation in Nursing) I sent to Esther saying that the package came from both Cynthia and me. Orlando knew I had lost contact with Cynthia and I suppose he assumed Esther knew that. Instead of treating it as a joke, his note hurt Esther deeply and she wrote and told her mother.

I knew nothing about my brother's joke until the day Esther's mother came to the hospital. Before I could greet her, she said, "I want to speak with you, Ben Sanidad."

"Of course," I said and wondered what I had done wrong.

As soon as we were alone, she said, "You are hurting my daughter's feelings." Then she started to cry.

I felt really scared then. I could not understand what I had done.

"Are you involved with Cynthia?" she asked.

"Hindi po!" (no ma'am in Filipino), I said.

Esther's mother stared into my eyes, but I was not sure she knew I was telling the truth. She did not say much more but when she left, she shook her finger at me and said, "Don't you hurt my daughter."

"I would not ever want to do that," I said. That evening I wrote to Esther and explained the best I could.

Apparently, Esther did not believe my explanation.

As a result of my brother's joke, we stopped writing for a few months and then only sporadically after that..

During those months, I felt lonelier than ever before. Her letters had taken my mind off my feelings of loneliness.

The intense loneliness returned.

Another thing I have to admit is that my quest for education never let up. As much as I cared about Esther, I cared more about my future than I did about her.

Eventually it became obvious that our relationship was over.

I found another girlfriend, but I never forgot Esther. It was over, I reminded myself many times.

If it was over, why did I constantly think of her?

\* \* \*

In 1971, after I had worked a full year with Dr. Fernando, he received a wonderful opportunity to study in California. He accepted the offer and took his family with him to Los Angeles.

I was happy for his opportunity. When anyone left the Philippines to become a doctor in the US they had to restart their medical education through a residency program. Despite being well known and already a gifted surgeon, like everyone else, he had to start again. He became a neuro-surgeon.

Esther was now a nurse working at White Memorial Medical Center in Los Angeles. She had her own apartment close to the hospital. Mrs.Fernando was also working there before her family arrived. Mrs. Fernando asked her if she could put up with her family until they found a place of their own.

"Of course, you may stay with me," Esther answered. Esther, even then, was a kind and generous person.

For almost a year, the Fernandos occupied her bedroom, and each night she slept in the living room or many times at her cousin Prescy's apartment.

Over the course of their living together, Esther got to know the Fernando family well. Somewhere during their many talks, Dr. Fernando told Esther about his niece Carol, a nurse at CVS. She was my girlfriend. I liked her, but not in any serious way.

I had become aware that some of the members of her family wanted me to marry her. The fact that I had never asked permission from her parents to date her should have told them that much. If I had had any serious thoughts of marriage, I would have taken that step as I had done with Esther's parents.

After Dr. Fernando met Esther and had lived with her a few months, he learned about us. Esther made it clear to him that even though we no longer corresponded regularly, she still cared deeply for me.

He wrote me a letter, and I do not remember his exact words, but it was obvious from the way he began that he believed I planned to marry Carol. In his letter he said that I should not marry Carol, and that he was convinced Esther was the woman for me. He closed his letter with these words, "Ben, if you are going to marry Carol, you are being blinded."

\* \* \*

Letters between Esther and me had become less frequent and much less passionate. Sometimes a month lapsed between responses. I did not realize Esther was pulling back because she thought I wanted to marry the other woman. Because I never mentioned Carol or wrote about dating her, she thought I was being deceptive. That strained our relationship even more.

Even though I cared about Esther, when I started to concentrate on getting to the US, I did not think about her as often or as deeply as I had before. My ambition took over and I allowed our relationship to disintegrate. My attention was focused on going to the US, and being accepted for internship or residency and begin somewhere by August of 1971.

The biggest hindrance for me was that the Philippine government required us to be accepted in a two-year residency program or a two-year service to the country before they allowed us to leave overseas for study. That meant I could do nothing until some school or government institution accepted me.

Every time I had a day off, which was about once a month, I took a bus to Manila and visited the Philippine government offices.

I went straight to the office and waited until they opened. My first priority was to check with them about the rules and regulations and then to apply again for release. I did not know what else to do.

By the time I had done five or six monthly trips, the clerks got to know me. I asked the same questions and made the same requests. They also gave me the same answers, but I persisted. It seemed to me that I was acting much like the widow in the biblical account of the unjust judge (*Luke 18*). The judge got so tired of the woman coming to see him that he finally settled her case to get her out of his sight.

Eventually, the clerks at the office must have realized how serious I was. Finally, one of them gave me a release form to apply for a student visa to go to the USA, even though I did not meet the requirements. Maybe, like the unjust judge, they just got tired of seeing my face and answering my questions again and again.

A few weeks after I started my work at CVS, Uncle Pros, another of mom's brothers, started his surgery residency in New York City. He wrote a letter that would soon open a door for me.

"There is an opening for surgical internship in my hospital. If you apply for it, there is a good chance that you can be admitted." He enclosed an application form for the Sydenhan City Hospital in Harlem.

Apparently the hospital had accepted an intern who backed out at the last minute. My uncle, who later became Chief surgical resident of the hospital, recommended me to his training professor—that he knew someone interested in the position, who was imminently qualified, and available.

The time seemed perfect. I was ready to go. The situation reminded me again of the saying, "It's whom you know and not what you know."

I filled out the form the same day I received it and mailed it back right away. Then I waited.

While eagerly waiting for a reply from New York, I continued to do my best work at CVS. Even though I wanted to go to the United States, I knew I was receiving absolutely the best training I could possibly get in the Philippines. During those days of waiting, I also took the qualifying examinations for US hospitals. Students could not just go and start their internship or residency. They first had to pass an examination for foreign medical graduates ECFMG (*Educational Council for Foreign Medical Graduates*). I took the exam and passed it. My having successfully completed that test, provided one of the tickets for me to go to the USA.

By the end of September, I left Manila by air. My dreams were starting to find fulfillment.

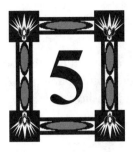

# A Twist of Events

*"And all things, whatsoever ye shall ask in prayer,
believing, ye shall receive."*
—Matthew 21:22 (KJV)

I began my internship at Sydenhan City Hospital, in Harlem. As I learned once I got there, that part of Harlem was a dangerous area with many drug addicts and homeless people roaming the streets.

The internship program demanded full concentration and left us little time for ourselves. I had to enroll in another internship program because U.S. hospitals did not recognize internship and residency programs in the Philippines and many other countries. For the first few months, I hardly had time to do anything of a personal nature. When I did, I was usually too tired and concentrated on catching up on my sleep.

Through mutual friends, Esther found out that I had come to the US, but she never wrote me in New York. I never wrote to tell her where I was. Our relationship had cooled off so much we had no contact. In fact, both of us probably thought our relationship was a thing of the past.

At first New York was wonderful. I had never seen such a large city before. It took awhile for me to learn to find my way around and get used to living in a different culture.

After a couple of weeks passed and I had barely adjusted to the new life, I began to feel lonely. I missed my friends in the Philippines. Somewhere during those cold, dark days of working in Harlem and having no social life, my thoughts turned again to Esther.

Was it possible we could get together? I asked myself that question many times, but I did nothing about it. After all, I had neglected her and because I felt guilty.I did nothing.

\* \* \*

In October 1971, Delma Quirante, a physician-friend of Uncle Pros and aunt Elma Lou planned to get married to Tony Chen, also a physician in Baltimore. She invited the family to the wedding. I think Uncle Pros knew how lonely I was and tried to help me adjust to my world.

"We'll drive up for the day," he said, "and be back by dark. Why don't you go along with us? It'll be good for you to get out of the city."

"Yes, I'd like to do that," I said. What I really meant was that I felt so lonely, I was glad to have an opportunity to go anywhere.

We drove to Baltimore early Sunday morning. Because we planned to change before the wedding, we wore casual clothes. When we reached the church, I slung the garment bag over my shoulder and followed my uncle and aunt inside.

Several people arrived at the same time. A young woman stood behind a table and held up a pen for newcomers to sign the guest book. She told the woman in front of me where she could change.

Just as my turn came and I reached out for the pen, I looked at her face. She was pretty and young, and she smiled at me. She wore a light-blue gown with a fragrant-smelling corsage around her neck.

I just stared at her and was shocked to see Esther. I was tongue-tied and unable to say a word.

I smiled at her and she smiled back!

We had not seen each other in six years. I paused, wanting to take in her features. She had changed a little, of course, and I decided she had become prettier than ever. Not sure what else to do, I reached out to shake her hand. Just then, memories of my behavior struck me. I felt ashamed and wanted to look away. Yet she smiled at me.

She giggled and held out her hand to shake mine. I took her hand, shook it, and I could not let go. I do not know why, but I held on as if I never wanted to let go. As I continued to stare at her, I kept thinking, you are so beautiful and sweet. I have missed you, really missed you. Finally, I let go of her hand.

I do not remember what we said to each other during the next few minutes, but when I walked away, the old flame of love had been rekindled. All sense of loneliness disappeared. Now finally, seeing Esther in person, I knew I really did love her.

It was a beautiful wedding, but I did not pay much attention to what went on. My mind had not left Esther. I wanted to know everything that had happened to her and to talk with her. Most of all, I wanted to find out if she still cared for me even a little. Was there someone else she cared about? Was she just being sweet because that was her job?

During the reception, as soon as she moved away from the rest of the wedding party, I walked over and said "hello" again. She smiled and answered as if we had seen each other only days before.

She is not angry, I thought. She does not hate me or want me to go away.

For the rest of the reception, I stayed close to Esther. With all the people moving around, chatting, introducing themselves, we still talked together as much as we could. In fact, having all those people milling around made it easier to keep the conversation light and friendly.

To my relief, Esther did not reproach me for the way I had treated her. In fact, she acted as if we had continued our romance by correspondence.

In my awkwardness, I kept saying something like, "It's a miracle, really a miracle that both of us are here today."

My life changed that day at the wedding. I knew—without the slightest doubt—that I loved Esther.

Uncle Pros must have sensed that we had reconnected. Two or three times he came by and said something in a light, teasing way about how nice we looked together, and how strange that we met again at a wedding.

Half an hour before the reception ended, Uncle Pros motioned for me to follow him so he could talk to me.

We moved to the opposite side of the room. With his back

toward her, he said, "I was thinking about Esther." He told me that he knew she had flown from Los Angeles to Baltimore and she had only a five-day vacation. From Baltimore, she was going to New York City to visit a friend. "You know, Ben, we could invite Esther to ride back to New York with us. What do you think of that?"

I was bashful and embarrassed, but I nodded and smiled. I could not think of anything I would rather have happen.

"Then ask her," he said.

I shook my head. "I—I can't." I had a lot of deep feelings, but I could not say anything to her of a personal nature.

"Do you want her to go with us?" he asked.

"Of course, but I—I can't ask her."

"Then I will," he said.

I watched from across the room while he walked over and talked to Esther. From there, I could not hear what they said, and I was too embarrassed to follow him and listen. My heart beat rapidly and my palms became moist during those few minutes. What if she refused? What if she did not want to see me again? What if she thinks I put Uncle Pros up to extending the invitation?

Just then Esther turned her head toward me and smiled at me from across the room. I smiled back. She was going to ride with us. I couldn't remember when I felt so happy.

\* \* \*

At the end of the reception came the big event when all the unmarried young women gathered and the bride tossed her bouquet. Esther caught it and everyone cheered.

Then all the single men lined up to catch the garter when the groom threw it. I caught it. I never did know if he had planned for me to get it since Esther got the bouquet and we had spent a lot of time together at the reception.

Everybody started to clap. "You're next," someone shouted at me. I am sure I blushed when everyone clapped for me after I caught the garter. The tradition said that whoever caught the flowers and the garter, were to be the next married. I do not know if we were the next couple to marry, but the rest of it was certainly true. Esther and I did marry.

## Memoir From the Groom, Tony . . .

I have a pretty good photographic memory of our first encounter.

Delma and I were married on October 10, 1971 in Baltimore, Maryland. Before the wedding day, Delma told me that she was playing cupid to reunite two lovebirds who were her friends. I had never met them before. She told me that Ben and Esther were in different parts of the US and that Ben had just arrived from the Philippines. She invited the two of them without them knowing that they would be under the same roof after a long period of separation from each other.

The moment I remembered most about Ben and Esther was at my wedding reception. Delma made sure that she threw the bouquet towards Esther who beat a lot of other ladies with her outstretched hand.

She whispered to me and pointed where Ben was standing in front of a bunch of enthusiastic young men who were waiting for the garter to be thrown. The pressure was on for both Ben and me. Quickly, I figured out a plan. I threw packets of sugar that I had hidden from the head table when my father-in-law was making the count to throw the garter. All the young men lunged for them and were distracted and disappointed. I then threw the garter towards Ben on the second count.

He really had to stretch out his hand to beat out the others.

Of course, there was a lot of clapping and also the tinkling sounds made by striking the glass with a metallic spoon. The waiters were startled, as they were not used to this tradition. Ben was ready to plant a kiss on his beloved Esther who was so shy and demure, tried to turn away her blushing face. Ben was such a romantic and gave Esther a good hug and a kiss.

Delma told me that was when the old flames were rekindled!

All of what I have described are on 8mm movies.

Finally, the wedding and reception were ended. We changed clothes once again. I remember waiting for Esther to come out. She wore a simple suit and looked as beautiful as if she wore an evening gown.

Uncle Pros led us all to the car. To my delight, aunt Elma Lou sat in the back of the Chevy station wagon. He had a bench seat in front so Esther and I could sit together for the five-hour trip to New York.

We had hardly gotten out of Baltimore when Uncle Pros said to Esther, "You need to help Ben a little."

"Help him to do what?"

"He's a lonely man. He wouldn't be so lonely if he had a pretty girl like you around."

Esther laughed.

"Yes, he goes to the hospital. He studies, eats and sleeps. That's all. I don't think that's healthy, do you?"

"No, he needs friends. He needs to do things." She said in her lovely cheerful voice.

"Maybe he needs to have people like you around so he can get out and enjoy himself."

"Maybe that's what he needs," she said.

The banter went on between them. From her face, I could tell that Esther enjoyed it as much as Uncle Pros.

I blushed a few times. Tried staring out the window, then at my hands or my feet.

I wanted to enter into the teasing, but I did not know what to say.

"I've been worried about Ben. When a man is lonely, he can find other women who are attractive. Yes, some are very, very attractive," Uncle Pros said. "A lot of women who don't belong to the Adventist church keep looking at him. I've seen them smiling and being nice to him,"

"Then if there are so many around, he shouldn't be lonely."

"But those women are not for Ben."

"But aren't there single women in the Adventist church in New York? I'm sure there are many—."

"They would be available, but they aren't what Ben needs, and

I've been concerned about him." Uncle Pros laughed and added, "I'm feeling better because you've come around."

I think Esther liked seeing me a little embarrassed and she did nothing to stop the teasing.

Uncle Pros told Esther about a Puerto Rican woman at the hospital. She seemed to like me, he told her. "And when she walks into the cafeteria, she sees only one person—our Ben."

"You had better keep a careful watch on him."

"It's nothing serious," I said. I explained that Carmelita and I had eaten lunch together several times in the cafeteria. I liked talking to her, but it has never been anything serious."

"Not serious for you, Ben," Uncle Pros said and laughed again. "But I have eyes too. I see the way she looks at my nephew."

Again, I felt embarrassed. Uncle Pros was right, and I did not realize he had observed her behavior. Carmelita had made it clear that she wanted to be more than just a friend. Although I never told Uncle Pros, the woman had begun to call me on the phone. Of course, it was flattering that she would do that, but it embarrassed me. Women had never called me before and in the Philippines, no woman would have done that.

Carmelita was a nice woman who went to church, but she was not an Adventist. That fact, more than anything else, bothered Uncle Pros. He was afraid I might be falling in love with her. In those days, very few people married outside our faith.

"I've been afraid he'd get involved with the wrong kind of woman," my uncle must have said to Esther at least four times. Other than a few observations and meeting her once, he did not know much about Carmelita. He did not have anything to say about her, but I think he told Esther so she would know that other women found me attractive.

* * *

After perhaps an hour, the joking between Uncle Pros and Esther finally stopped. Esther and I started talking to each other a little, but I did not say much. Being in the car with my uncle and aunt made it easier in some ways. Both of us knew we could not say anything particularly personal to each other.

It was also hard, because I wanted to hold her hand. Not only was I too shy to do that, but also with my uncle in the front seat with us, I just could not feel comfortable even sitting close to Esther.

For most of the rest of the trip, I sat quietly and listened. Obviously, my uncle and Esther liked each other. With their talking and laughing, no one paid much attention to me, and that helped me feel less embarrassed.

Finally, we reached Manhattan, where Esther's friend, Jedd Santos-Villanueva lived. Before she got out of the car, I did have the courage to ask Esther for her phone number.

She smiled and took out a piece of paper and wrote it down for me.

Nothing else happened, but I knew we had reconnected. I knew I cared, but I was still afraid that Esther did not feel as strongly as I did.

* * *

The next morning I went to work, but I could not concentrate. No matter what was going on, my thoughts kept turning to Esther. I wanted to see her again. About the middle of the morning, I talked to Uncle Pros and told him how I felt.

"Then you must see her."

"But what should I do? I don't have any money to take her—."

He laid his hand on my shoulder. "I'll take care of that. Why don't you call around the city and see if there's anything going on that you'd like to take Esther to?"

Before I could protest about money, he said, "I'll pay for the entertainment." He slapped me on the shoulder and said, "We can't let Esther get lonely while she's in New York, can we?"

I made a few calls, found out about a Broadway musical program at Radio City. Because I was sure she would like it, I called her. When she said she would like to go with me, I told Uncle Pros and he bought our tickets.

"Esther is the one for you," my uncle said. "Yes, definitely, she is the one for you."

He was right, of course, and I was too bashful to tell him I already knew that.

# A Twist of Events

* * *

We had a really nice time at Radio City. For the first time we talked—the way we had opened ourselves to each other through our letters. The shyness vanished and I felt comfortable in talking to Esther.

Before I took Esther to Jedd's apartment, I invited her to visit Sydenhan City Hospital. I wanted her to come, but I felt a lot of concern about her safety, because of its location in a rough part of Harlem. In those days, it was dangerous for strangers to walk around. Drug addicts and street people were everywhere at any time of the day or night. Sometimes people were mugged.

To my delight, Esther did visit me at the hospital. Once there, she agreed it was not the best environment to work in. I felt so grateful that she would come. I proudly introduced her to everyone I knew.

I took off as much time as I could during the next few days, which was mostly only an hour or two a day. I enjoyed the few things we were able to do together. Whenever I had free time I called her. No, it was not a lot of time, but during those four days we talked about us, about the past, about our future dreams, but neither of us mentioned marriage.

During those days, I kept trying to push from my mind that she'd be gone soon.

Then she was gone. As I said good-bye to her at the airport, I thought, I have just found her again and now she is going back to California.

After Esther returned to California, we began to write to each other again. Our letters went out the same day we received them, just as they had done in the Philippines. This time we had the added advantage of the telephone, although I seldom could afford to call.

As I learned later, Esther was not very interested in pursuing a relationship with me at first, because she still thought I was interested in Dr. Fernando's niece. Her letters were friendly, but they lacked the warmth we had shared before. Once she realized that there was nothing between Carol and me, she warmed up. The letters began to sound like the Esther of old. And I realized how much I had missed writing to her.

Our telephone conversations became more frequent. Esther has always been a generous person. In those days, she freely spent the money to call me or we would have had few telephone conversations. She had a job with money coming in; I was living on a small stipend and had to be very careful with every cent. She understood my situation.

It would have hurt my pride to have her pay for the calls except that both of us knew it was only temporary. I also knew I could not let her out of my life again.

\* \* \*

We had rekindled such a good relationship, even though her receptive response had rather stunned me. I realized later, that in the beginning of our getting back together, she was not really serious about me. Maybe it was a matter of trust; she may have been afraid of being hurt by me again. She was not convinced there was no one else in my life.

Although I did not know it then, Uncle Pros, convinced that God wanted Esther and me to marry, called her several times. The most important call came when he said, "Ben needs to buy a car. But in order for him to get a good one, he needs $500 for a down payment.

"Yes, I can do that," Esther said.

She did not realize what Uncle Pros was doing. When Esther called and offered me a loan, I did not figure it out either. My uncle could have loaned me the money himself.

I bought the car—a new 1972 Ford Grand Torino. Having my own car made life easier, and I was grateful to Esther.

\* \* \*

Our telephone calls went on almost every evening I was off or during the day when I had night duties. We talked and talked. I was so lonely in New York and looked forward to her calls as the best part of my day. So many times I would come to the quarters tired and drained, and that was when I felt the loneliest. Then the phone would ring and it would be Esther. Just listening to her soft, cheerful voice made me feel better. As I often told her, her calls inspired me to get up and work hard the following day.

Each day I became more convinced that I wanted to marry her

and finally asked her to marry me.

"Yes, I'll marry you," Esther answered, "and I love you."

Those were the most wonderful words I could have heard.

We set the date to get married: September 24, 1972.

Matthew 21:22 reads, "And all things, whatsoever ye shall ask in prayer, believing, ye shall receive." The fervent prayers of our parents in our behalf would soon come to realization.

# Marriage and Career

*"Wives, submit yourselves unto your own husbands, as unto the Lord."*—Ephesians 5:22 (KJV)

*"Husbands, love your wives, even as Christ also loved the church, and gave himself for it."*—Ephesians 5:25 (KJV)

*"And unto the married I command, let not the wife depart from her husband."*—1 Corinthians 7:10 (KJV)

For a long time—since I was eight years old—I had dreamed about becoming a surgeon. It was the only form of medicine I thought about.

It was a dream that would never become a reality.

I had arrived too late to begin my internship in New York. One year—one full year—that was the rule and there was no way the hospital would allow me to cut the time short. Because I had to complete a full year, I would not be ready for my residency in October of 1972.

Unfortunately for me, residency training in the US schools begins in June or July. When all the residency programs began in the summer, I still had three months to stay at Sydenhan City Hospital in Harlem. If I pursued my dream to become a surgeon, I would have to apply to hospitals to take me and then wait for nine months to get into the next program.

While doing my internship at Sydenhan, I did apply for several residency programs in surgery. Even though I knew it was not likely, I still hoped—and I even prayed—that I would find an opening just as I had for my internship. No doors opened, no programs had vacancies.

I felt discouraged and unsure what I should do. I could try to find a job, such as working in an emergency room while waiting for the program to start. It was not what I wanted to do, but I was willing—anything to have money coming in while I waited for an opening.

Then suddenly there was a residency opening. The sad news was that the opening was not in the surgery department. I faced a serious dilemma. I had to make a choice—one that would decide what my career in medicine would be.

Aunt Elma Lou was an anesthesiology resident in St. Luke's Hospital in Manhattan. One man backed out in her program three months into his residency, which left an empty slot. She asked me if I was interested in being an anesthesiologist. "If you are," she said, "I'm sure I can help you get it."

"I'm interested," I said, "but I need to think about it."

"I understand. It's a big decision for you."

She knew my dream had always been to be a surgeon. If I accepted the residency in anesthesiology, that dream would end.

For two days, I gave it a lot of serious thought. Of course, I prayed for God's help in making the decision, but it was more a matter of going through a ritual. I did not expect any kind of direction from God. I received no answer from God either.

After waiting for another six months, until June or July, what if I still don't land a job? Then for half a year, I will have nothing to do. I thought about having no money coming in as well. I would have to do something to support myself for those months of waiting. Even if I chose to wait, I had no assurance that I would be accepted in any surgical residency program. If I said yes to anesthesiology, there would be no turning back. I would say goodbye to my childhood dreams. But if I said yes, I could still be in medicine. That also meant I could start my final training right away. I could not wait.

"I might as well accept the residency training in anesthesia," I told aunt Elma Lou.

She smiled. We talked quite a while but I think she had known when she told me about the program that I would eventually say yes.

The next day, I applied, was interviewed, and they accepted me.

It was a two-year program with an option of taking a third year.

At last, my dreams were finally becoming reality.

\* \* \*

After I finished my internship on September 15, 1972, I drove my Ford Grand Torino to Southern California to see Esther. We were married September 24, 1972. Of course, I thought it was the most beautiful wedding I had ever seen.

Esther had planned it well, and everything went without problems. It was a happy and joyous occasion, and it became especially wonderful because more than 500 people attended. That number included both our relatives, but most of them were Esther's friends. It reminded me of what a warm, friendly person she was, because so many came to her special day.

Esther's father, an SDA minister, came from the Philippines to give the hand of his daughter to me. The following day, we rented a U-Haul trailer and pulled it behind the Grand Torino. We were going back to New York. As a honeymoon, Esther and I took six days to travel across the country to New York.

We arrived at our apartment on Sunday night—a one-bedroom apartment I had rented just before I drove to California. It was comfortable and across the street from the hospital. It was not spacious or outstanding, but it was inexpensive. Despite the small space, both of us knew we would only have to live there a couple of years.

Monday morning I started my residency program in anesthesia. Esther applied and was hired for a nursing position at the Woman's Hospital, located next to St. Luke's. She worked until our first child was born, June 15, 1973. We named him Benjamin Sanidad III.

\* \* \*

I finished my residency in anesthesiology September 30, 1974. Before the end of my two-year residency I started applying for a place to work and visited hospitals in New York, New Jersey, Maryland, Pennsylvania and other places in the South. Again I found difficulty in finding a place that would take me as the open slots had already been filled up by anesthesiologists who finished their residency months before I did.

In the meantime, the residency director offered me the option to start the third year program specializing in Open Heart Anesthesia. He gave me the choice to either continue in the program until I was able to find a job or to finish the optional third-year residency program.

I gave it a lot of consideration, but I had worked and studied a lot of years. I wanted to get out on my own and do what I had been trained to do if there was a job offer.

In November 1974, I received a job offer—my first. A hospital medical director in Big Springs, Texas, about two hundred miles south of Dallas, contacted me.

By now I could hardly wait to get out of New York City. The size, the crowded conditions, the fast pace of the city was more than I wanted. I wanted to raise my family in a smaller community and among neighbors I could get to know.

I decided to go out to Texas and look it over. Esther and I agreed that if I liked the place, I would say yes.

In the meantime, a Filipino friend named Dr. Samuel Lardizabal contacted me. He was an anesthesiologist in Marion, Ohio, which is fifty miles north of Columbus. "I want you to come to Marion, Ben, because I'm ready to expand my practice," he told me, "and I want a partner."

Sam wanted me badly enough that he set up a deal. Instead of my buying into the business, if I came, he would make me a partner and I would receive $45,000 a year, which was what they offered me in Texas without a partnership.

After getting by for years on a fraction of that amount, either offer seemed like a lot of money. I was not sure I wanted to move to Ohio, since I had never been there. Because of its location, maybe I thought it was too close to New York. I was not sure why I wanted to go to Texas. Maybe it was the lure of the west and the mental image of what Texas was supposed to be like. We had driven through the panhandle on our honeymoon and the people had been quite friendly. I liked the rural scenes we had driven past.

I really made my mind to go to Texas. Sam did not give up, however. He called me regularly. "Just come and visit. See what we have to offer here," he would say.

"Okay, I'll fly out there and see how it is before I make up my mind," I told him.

I never got out of New York. On the date I was to go, I was driving to La Guardia airport. On the way, the car in front of me suddenly stopped. To avoid an accident, I threw on my brakes, but the car behind me did not stop fast enough. He rear-ended me. I ended up with whiplash that was so severe, the pain would not allow me to do anything except lie in bed.

A week later, I rescheduled my trip to Ohio. At that point, going to Marion, Ohio, was more an act of courtesy than anything else because Sam was an old friend.

I visited Marion in January, nine months before I would finish my third year residency program. I can not explain it, but when I went around Marion, I absolutely loved the place. It was cool, but not as cool or as overcast as I was used to seeing in January in New York. The clean streets amazed me—nothing like what I had seen in Harlem. People spoke or smiled, most of the time before I did. I met the doctors Sam worked with. All of them seemed friendly. I did not feel that frosty reserve so common to New York.

I knew I had found my place. "You've won me over," I told Sam.

Immediately, I telephoned Esther. "We're moving to Ohio," I said. To Esther, it did not matter where we moved. We were a family and we would be together and soon have our own home. She was elated.

I told my residency program director about the job offer.

"Take the partnership," he said. "You're ready. This is a better move for you."

* * *

We rented a Ryder truck and drove from New York to Ohio in February 1975. Esther had no adjustment problem. She loved Marion because it was a beautiful town—not far from a large city, but small enough that she felt we could raise a family there. She had lived in the crowded cities of Los Angeles and New York. Now she was ready for Marion.

Somehow, both of us knew Marion, Ohio, was going to be

home for us for a long, long time.

\* \* \*

While I was finishing my residency in New York, I went to Virginia to take the Federal Licensing Examination Program or FLEX. It was an examination for the states that had a reciprocal licensing agreement. Virginia had reciprocity with the nearby states around us, such as Ohio and New York. Texas also recognized it and so did most states.

I passed the FLEX, applied for a New York license, and it was granted. I also applied for both Ohio and Texas. Both of them would grant me a license, but I never did follow up with Texas.

There was just one problem. For some reason unknown to me, it takes months for reciprocating states to issue a license. When I went to Ohio the first week in February, I still did not have a license to practice in that state.

I learned that Dr. Frederick Merchant, chairman of FLEX, had a surgical practice right at Marion General Hospital. When I arrived, they needed me badly as an anesthesiologist. So Dr. Merchant wrote to the Ohio board. Instead of waiting two or three months, within a week I had my license to practice in Ohio.

\* \* \*

Once we moved to Ohio, I joined Sam with a one-year contract as his partner. Although Sam and I liked each other very much and we had no personal problems, after a few months, I realized I did not like our business relationship.

I worked extremely hard and put in an uncountable number of hours. Regardless of how hard I worked—and I did not know how not to work hard—I still made $45,000. I felt as if I deserved to make more. Our agreement was such that I was free to leave any time and set up my own practice.

At Marion General Hospital, they have four operating rooms. When I arrived, Sam was the chairman of the anesthesiology department, and he decided which rooms we anesthesiologists would take. In those days, besides Sam and me, there were two others. I may have been mistaken, but it seemed to me that he always chose the best

71

rooms and best patients for himself—those who were elective cases and who were healthy and young. They required less work.

That inequity caused friction between us. I insisted that all four of us should function on the same level. "Give everyone an equal share of easy and difficult surgeries."

Sam did not agree with me. He also did not agree with me on the assignment method, which was under his control.

The biggest issue, however, continued to be over money. I did not find it satisfying to work under him for a set salary. Whether I worked hard or got as much surgery as I could, my salary remained the same. We talked about it, and I realized Sam was not going to change.

I decided to go on my own, but I stayed with the partnership until I had finished my one-year agreement. We parted on good terms.

I established my own practice in 1976, which was, of course, more profitable for me. I worked hard and tried to be available any time for my patients. Here is an example of how it became more profitable to me. One doctor might decide to handle only three cases in one day because he did not want to work long hours. I might take five, which was almost like doing a double shift. Sometimes the others would ask me to accept weekend call when it was their duty. Whenever I could, I agreed. Because I was then being paid by each case I took, my income rose steadily.

\* \* \*

When we arrived in Marion, one of the first things Esther asked was, "Where's the nearest church?" By that, she meant a Seventh-day Adventist church. We found a small one in the city, joined it, and became members.

Shortly after we joined, they invited me to become an officer, but I declined, citing my busy schedule. That was not the real reason, but it satisfied them. It also explained when I did not attend church very often.

By 1975, when we moved to Ohio, nothing about worship and Bible study excited me, and I often found it boring. Esther, however, was far more spiritual, and the church became a vital part of her life. When the children came along, she took them to church on Sabbath and other church and youth activities.

We soon had a lovely family with three children. Besides Ben, who was born in New York in 1973, Nicholette, whom we have always called Nikki, was born in Ohio in October 1975. The following year, Gaylord was born, but he took my family nickname and has always been called Arti.

When they grew up, they eventually became school leaders in their respective classes.

* * *

Sam, my former partner, decided to move to California. That gave me even more opportunities. I stayed busier than before. Money seemed to pour in, even though I worked hard for it. I kept reminding myself that I lived a totally happy life. Some days I even believed it—when I was not too busy working.

Occasionally, I took vacations with my family. I did love them and wanted to promote a good family life. As I look back, I sincerely believe that despite my selfishness and lack of concern about God, Esther and my children knew I loved them and cared very much about them.

Even though I sometimes felt guilty about it, I had no interest in the church and could not seem to find any reason to get interested. I went to church and promised myself that I would attend regularly and get involved. I kept finding excuses not to attend. I made sure I was on call most Saturdays, and that kept me out of church most weeks.

Besides, going to church began to seem like a waste of time. I saw no particular need to change my life. After all, anyone could look at me and know that I was a good man with a moral background. When I examined my life—which was not often—I felt I had everything I needed. Church and God were all right, they just were not important.

Before long, I became head of the Anesthesiology Department, a position I held for several years. It gave me the opportunity to invite other anesthesiologists to join me. When they came in, their salary was based on the amount of work they actually did. We had a really good working relationship. By then, Marion had six anesthesiologists, and four were in my practice. There was enough work for all of us.

Everything in my life was going well. I was making far more

money than I had ever dreamed of. I invested carefully and my investments paid off. I was living what some would call a charmed life.

That was all outward. Inwardly, dissatisfaction had begun to grow. Because I did not understand it, I did not know how to handle it. I knew only that I did not like my life very much and I did not know why or what to do.

It was not my work, because I enjoyed that immensely. I loved my family. If I took my life one item at a time and examined it, I liked everything. But I still felt something was missing. At times I became aware of an emptiness I could not explain, and I certainly could not talk about it, not even to Esther.

I wanted something more—something else that would excite me. I needed variety, something to challenge me. But I had no idea what that something else was.

As a child in the Philippines I had wanted to become a pilot. Maybe, I thought, if I became a pilot, that would fill the empty spaces. After considering that idea for several days, I enrolled in a flying school in Marion.

As often as possible, I took the lessons. Several times I turned down opportunities to do extra work at the hospital. I had a new goal and it did invigorate me. Within six months, I went solo. That was not enough. I kept at it until I passed my test and received a pilot's license. Then I bought my own plane, a Cessna 150.

I thoroughly enjoyed flying short distances around Ohio on my days off. I was alone in the clouds, with my own plane. No one else was around, and I felt contentment—for a while.

Then the feeling of emptiness crept back in. Why am I doing this? I asked myself. Is this all there is to life? If I am so successful, why I do not feel happy? Learning to fly had only temporarily hidden the emptiness. I had only been kidding myself.

I could not stand the feeling of worthlessness, of emptiness, of wanting something more out of life and not knowing what it was. If it ever occurred to me to stop and examine my life or to turn to God, I was not listening. I kept looking "out there" for a solution.

I had to try something else. I decided to join the U.S. Air Force Reserve. No one had to recruit me—I was searching for something to bring excitement into my life. Normally, the federal government offered nice sums of money as incentives. I did not ask or receive any special benefits; I simply joined the Air Force.

Esther, always supportive of me, agreed when I said I wanted to join the Reserves. Because of her exposure to United States Clarkfield Air Force Base in the Philippines, she had a positive attitude toward the Air Force.

Did she sense what I was going through? I did not ask. I kept thinking that something was wrong with me and I had to find a way to fix myself. Maybe the military was the fix I needed.

The Air Force commissioned me as a Major. Once I became a reserve, I had to spend one weekend a month on reserve duty. I was trained as what they called a flight surgeon. I never operated on anyone and the title was misleading. Mostly, I made sure that pilots were physically fit to fly. I flew with them, which was what I wanted to do.

As a flight surgeon, I enjoyed the job immensely. It seemed like the answer I had been seeking.

For a while.

Esther was busy raising our three children and remained heavily involved in the church and community. Saying nothing and not object- ing to my decisions was the way she had been brought up. She had been only seventeen years old when she moved to the United States. The influence of the church taught her that she was to love and to sup- port her husband.

If I had been true to my background as a Filipino, I would have been so involved with my family that I would have asked their per- mission before I took flying lessons and especially before I joined the reserves. After I came to the United States, however, I realized that most American men—at least those I knew and worked with—did not do things that way. It did not take me long to learn that they decided what they wanted to do, told their wives and family, and then they did it. That is how I behaved—not really concerned about the family.

By 1990, I was living the good life, according to all my friends and colleagues. I had my own plane, was an Officer in the Air Force Reserves, and our office had as much work as we could handle. For several years, I had carefully invested in property and made money on it. I bought sports cars and even a boat. We had a beautiful vacation home on a lake fifty miles from Marion. Everywhere I looked everything seemed just about perfect.

Despite all the empty feelings inside—and they continued to grow—I never thought about God. Instead, I tried to find happiness in all these material things.

Then came the Persian Gulf War, when Americans and other nations sent troops into the Desert Storm War. My call came in January of 1991. I had been activated.

Frankly, I was delighted. I did not want to kill people, but I wanted to be on the scene where things were happening and people were feeling challenged and excited.

## *Esther's Reflections....*

When President George Bush declared war with Iraq, I watched the news so much which I had never done before, especially when he said more troops would be activated. I kept asking myself, "Will Ben be next?"

The following day after Ben came home from work, we decided to go out shopping to buy shoes for him. My thoughts at all times were about the war and the possibility that Ben may be called to serve the country. When we came back home, we got a message from Kathy, my secretary that Ben was to report for duty right away at the U.S. Air Force base in Springfield, Ohio.

After hearing the message, I felt as if a whole mountain dropped over me. I hugged my husband and cried. When my children came home from school, I told them the news and they also cried. Things after that just went very fast.

Many questions kept popping up in my mind like, "What if I will never see him again?" "How can I take care of my children alone?" "How about his office?"

Before leaving for Springfield, he decided to walk our kids to school, then on our way to the Base, Ben talked to me about the office and things I needed to do in his absence.

In one room at the Base, I met many nervous and fearful

wives, lawyers, and chaplains. One chaplain gave me a small Bible. Then, a lot of paper signing . . ., like power of attorney, etc. I felt I was giving up and surrendering my husband to the government. I had mixed feelings. I was happy for him to serve the country but sad and confused not knowing if I will ever see him again alive.

The first month after he left, I was feeling down and lonely, wanting to sleep all the time. I spent my waking hours lying down in bed staring at the ceiling or watching the news, and only to come back out to cook food for my children. Office papers were strewn all over the room. Finally, our children encouraged me to start getting out and doing other things. I knew they were right.

One Sabbath day, my children and I were invited for lunch at our aunt and Uncle Tangunan's place. My uncle asked me if I would say grace before the meal. I thanked God for the delicious food and also asked God that the war would end soon and wanted for Ben to come home.

That prayer was answered! The following day, President Bush declared the war was over. I was joyful and ecstatic!

The Air Force sent me to Cannon Air Force Base in Arizona. Once I got there, I learned they did not need an anesthesiologist. I was transferred to the Nellis Air Force Base in Las Vegas, Nevada where an anesthesiologist was needed to help re-open the hospital surgery department. Most of the hospital doctors and nurses had gone to the Middle East.

I was willing to go or do whatever the Air Force asked, but I had really wanted to go to the Middle East.

When I arrived at Nellis, other reserve doctors had already reported for duty. We had to work hard and quickly to get things going. In one week we started doing surgeries again. During that time, they also started to train us to take over in the Middle East if we were needed. The Gulf War lasted only a few weeks. Had it lasted months, I would have gone overseas.

By the end of May 1991, the Air Force released me and I returned to Ohio. I had not closed the practice, and everything was ready for me to step right back into things as they had been.

Is that what I wanted? I asked myself that several times. During those weeks away, I had changed. I did not know what happened, but I knew I was different. I felt as if I had nothing in common with my partners in the office. One by one, I had released them to start their own independent practice. We cooperated, but they no longer worked for me. I had started the process about a year before the Gulf War. I think that even then I was preparing to make changes, to get away, to do something different. I did not want to feel responsible for them.

Because I had been in the community many years and was liked and respected, it was no problem to pick up my practice again. And I did. Business was as good as ever. Success smiled on me everywhere I looked.

Then "why don't I feel happy and successful? Why don't I enjoy my life more? What am I missing?"

I was not ready to know the answer. It would take a long time and a serious illness to make me answer my own question.

I kept thinking, I work hard in the hospitals and Esther works hard in the community. We are doing all the right things. In fact, Esther received the Golden Heart Award. It was a very prestigious award given in Marion for those who did the most to help the poor and disadvantaged.

Esther got me involved, and I did what she asked. Even though she tried hard to involve me and I cooperated, in my mind it was Esther's project and I supported her.

It worked this way. Esther became concerned about the poor and their need for affordable housing. One day she was driving and saw a badly run-down house for sale. She looked it over and saw that, with a few hundred dollars, it could be repaired and made livable for a family.

She asked me to buy it and I did, and I also paid for the repairs. Once it was ready, she worked with a community organization and we sold it to a low-income family without interest, and for less than the house was actually worth. Once they paid for the house, it was theirs. We took their payments and bought another, run-down-but-repairable house. Over a period of a couple of years, we bought, repaired, and sold three houses. Esther felt it was a way we could help people who needed help. I did not object, but I never got emotionally involved the way she did.

By the early 1990s our children were growing up, and I wanted to spend more time with them. Maybe that would revitalize me. As I became more involved, I realized how little we had done together in their growing-up years. We had taken family vacations, that kind of thing, but I wanted to bond with my children. So I decided to find ways to join them in their activities.

All three of my kids sing, and they joined a singing group, Rainbow Express, that performed in different churches in and around Marion. I supported them morally and financially and, as much as possible, I attended their singing engagements.

When my kids took up golf, I took up golf too. When they tried roller blading or scuba diving, I joined them. I had not done any of those things before, but I was still young enough to learn, and I did. To my surprise, I really enjoyed doing the fun things with them.

In all those years I never thought much about my health. I abused my body by overeating and not exercising regularly—the two most obvious things—but I did not think about what I was doing.

My eating patterns were terrible. I ate anything I wanted. I had been brought up to believe that a non-meat diet is better, but I had ignored all I knew about nutrition. My body ballooned. I am a short man anyway, and the weight made me look even shorter.

Then came the day when my body rebelled. That was when I stared at death and it scared me.

# A Life or Death Crisis

*"Then shall ye call upon me, and ye shall go and pray unto me, and I will hearken unto you. And ye shall seek me and find me when ye shall search for me with all your heart."*
—Jeremiah 29:12-13 (KJV)

"What do you want me to do, Lord?"

Just before I turned fifty-one, those words were the most honest I had spoken to God in my life. For several days, I continued to ask the question because I did not know where else to turn in my bewilderment.

I needed help, and yet I could not explain what was wrong. So I simply said, "What's next God?" I prayed those words sincerely in moments of what some might call quiet desperation. It was not that I never prayed to Him. It was more that God was not the focus of my life.

What probably brought the question into focus was an awareness that I had been dividing my life into five-year periods. At the end of each, I made a drastic change. For instance, in 1990, I joined the Air Force. After the Gulf War, I got out of the Air Force Reserve in 1995 as a Lt. Colonel. As I faced 1996, I asked myself, "What is ahead for me during the next five years?" It was more than just making a change. Although I did not grasp it then, that prayer was a deep-felt cry of desperation, a way of asking, "How do I find meaning in my life?"

"What am I going to do now?"

"I have everything in life I need. My wife is faithful and loving. Our kids have grown up to be good, healthy, and loving. What do you want me to do?"

No answer came. Maybe I was not ready for an answer. Maybe God had to show me in a more dramatic way before I would listen. And God did show me.

* * *

On March 30, four days after my birthday, I fainted in the operating room.

Once I knew it was esophageal cancer, I did not question it. I accepted the inevitable. And accepting it meant that my life was over.

My colleagues urged me to have surgery, but I kept thinking, it does not make any difference, because I'm not going to survive. That kind of thinking made me decide to do whatever my doctors advised and also not wanting to disappoint them—trying so hard to help.

All right," I said, "I'll do whatever you say."

* * *

Dr. Christopher Ellison scheduled my surgery for 8:00 AM, Monday, April 8. After visiting his office, I immediately returned home and I did the obvious and sensible thing: I closed my office.

My feelings? I was distraught, depressed and terrified. Twenty years of medical practice and the role suddenly changed. My future: uncertain and bleak.

Then my life took a second turn—and at last, it was the right way to turn. I can not explain all the reasons, only to say that I began to pray and to read the Bible. I realized as I lay in the quietness of our bedroom that I was alone. Yet not really alone, only unaware. God had been reaching out to me all my adult life, but I had ignored those loving hands.

It may sound strange, but the hardest part was that I did not know how to approach the Lord in those first hours. I just said, "Lord, I am sick. What will you have me to do now? Will you allow me to die? Will you allow me to suffer?"

"Your way is the only way," I said, and as I spoke those words, I knew they were true.

"I have to touch the hand of the Lord," I kept thinking. "He is waiting for me. He is calling to me and now I have to turn."

"God, please, please help me. Lord, I can't do anything without

81

you." That was a totally new experience to me. My parents had tried to implant in me the love of God. In some vague way, I knew that God loved me, and I did not doubt it. I prayed to him as I had been taught, but I did not really feel him or think much about God. This time it was different.

Praying wore me out and sapped my strength, but I did not give up. Finally, in my weariness, I said, "Lord, it's not my will now. It's your will, reveal your will to me."

God began to transform me and my entire view of life started to change. At first, I did not know how to talk to Esther about my new-found faith, but I did not need to say much. She saw it happening and encouraged me.

During those days I also thought of our three children. I wanted to draw close to my family. Ben had married and lived in Mount Vernon, Ohio; Nikki and Arti were in school near Chattanooga, Tennessee, at Southern Adventist University. I wanted to see them, talk to them, and express my love for them.

Esther called them home. For the previous six months, it had been only Esther and me alone.

But I would not be alone and separated anymore. As long as God gave me life, I would draw closer to Esther and to our children and to Jesus Christ.

Then I would never feel alone again.

# Making the Choice

*"Hear me when I call, O God of my righteousness: thou hast enlarged me when I was distressed; have mercy upon me and hear my prayer."*—Psalms 4:1(KJV)

"No, I won't accept that you will die," Esther said. "I will do my best to keep you alive with the help of the Lord." Those sounded like strange words to me in 1996. What could Esther do? The best doctors in the country had examined me. Surgery had already been scheduled in a few days, followed by chemotherapy and radiation, and in a few months I would die.

At first, I thought those were only the words of a loving, caring wife who would not surrender to the inevitable. She meant more than that.

"We can fight this together," she insisted. "Don't give up."

Her words gave me a renewed spirit. Esther was determined to get help that would keep me alive. She showed me that she was really behind me. She contacted all the members of my family as well as my parents who now lived in Toronto. She thought that having them close would raise my spirits and help me to fight harder. She called people in our church and every local pastor she knew to ask for their prayers. Over the next few days, she called Adventist pastors in other parts of the country. Every day, she would think of someone else. When she contacted them, she urged them to pray for me.

I received support from the hospital—the nurses, doctors, and other staff people—as well as church members. Theresa Hunt a lovely lady who works in the operating room, Carver Williams, Chaplain,

Lisa Cudd, Gayle and Gary Holback, Janet and Burt Patterson, Chris Sobas and Pastor Walter Arties, Voice of Prophecy director of Evangelism, were some of the people who constantly kept in touch and prayed for me and my family.

To my surprise, when former patients heard that I had cancer, they started sending notes and calling me. The prayers at my home began on Tuesday evening. Wednesday, people visited at all hours. The phone rang constantly. People—many of them strangers— wanted to pray for me and to express their concern. Thursday and Friday, relatives came to see me from California, Virginia, Canada, and Chicago. It amazed me to see the love, care and concern people showed.

Saturday night my wife called an anointing service for me. Esther believed the words of James 5:14-15 (*KJV*): "Are any among you sick? They should call for the elders of the church, and have them pray over them, anointing them with oil in the name of the Lord. And their prayer offered in faith will heal the sick, and the Lord will make them well. And anyone who has committed sins will be forgiven."

In our living room, my family, relatives and close friends sang hymns and prayed while the anointing service was going on.

I knelt in my bedroom surrounded by Pastor Raj Attiken, currently President of the Ohio SDA Conference, Pastor Rom, our church Pastor, my father, my Uncle Peter Roda, an anesthesiologist from Hinsdale, and my father-in-law, Pastor Ignacio Hernando, Sr.

They laid their hands on my head while they prayed. Suddenly, I felt as though an electric current from heaven surged through my whole body through their warm hands. I also felt peace. I did not experience any physical kind of feeling, but I felt my faith grow within me. It was what I called a renewed spirit.

For the first time since I had learned of the cancer, I began to hope. I knew the Lord was with me.

"Maybe...maybe I can survive," I thought.

I had always feared death. I had seen many people who experienced unbearable pain before they died. I was terrified and it frightened me to think of my own painful death. But after those church leaders prayed, I was comforted and my faith strengthened. Their supplications in my behalf gave me assurance of a possible healing. James 5:16 (*KJV*) say, "Pray one to another, that ye may be healed." I claimed this promise.

Before surgery, I underwent a lot of tests; mostly blood tests and a CAT (*Computed Axial Tomography*) scan. They found a lesion in my liver, which indicated that the cancer had already spread. However, when Dr. Ellison saw the pictures, he said, "I don't think this is cancer."

I also underwent nuclear medicine tests. They tried to tag the dyes and find out whether the lesion absorbed the dye or not. Fortunately, it did not, which indicated that the lesion was not cancerous. The doctor decided it was a benign tumor of the vessels, a hemangioma.

Before I went into surgery, Dr. Ellison clearly explained to Esther and me what would happen. If he found the cancer had spread beyond the esophagus, he would not operate but recommend chemotherapy and radiation. If the growth had not spread, he would totally resect (cut) the esophagus, that is, take out my esophagus and a part of my stomach. What is left of the stomach would be pulled up and connect to my throat to make a new esophagus.

Monday morning the scope test was done.

\* \* \*

When I awakened that afternoon, I did not know what had happened. I felt my throat, but I could not move very much. My breathing was controlled by a machine and I had tubes in my mouth and nostrils. I felt so weak, but the presence of tubes told me what I needed to know. They had operated on me.

"Ah, that means the cancer hasn't spread," I thought. Just knowing that much added another ray of hope. The cancer had not spread. It was just possible I would survive.

Immediately after surgery, Dr. Ellison came out of the operating room and told my family that he found positive lymph nodes.

My wife and children decided that I would not be told about the findings, because they felt I might feel discouraged and would give up while I was still in a critical situation.

* * *

The day after surgery, Dr. Ellison came to visit me.

"I did biopsies of the lymph nodes, Ben," he said, "I removed three lymph nodes and two are positive."

Those words burst my balloon of hope. Depression swept over me.

After he left, I wondered why he had operated. He had said that if it had spread, he would close me up. But he had not done that. He had operated. Did that mean he thought I might survive after all?

We never talked about it, but I began to believe that when my doctor did not find anything in the scope, he went ahead and operated. He removed the lesion on the esophagus. And while he was operating, he discovered the lymph nodes and removed as many as he could.

The next morning, Wednesday, the doctor said, "We're going to prepare you for chemotherapy and radiation to fight the cancer cells that are still there."

From those words and the other things he said, I knew he was almost a hundred percent sure there were still cancer cells there.

So I am going to die, I thought. I will go for chemotherapy and radiation, but it won't make any difference.

It is strange, because I am not a person who easily gives up. But when it came to my life, it was different. I am a medical man. If one of my colleagues—especially one considered the best—says "It's cancer," that is the verdict.

## *Esther's Reflections...*

I thought I was calm and could handle the situation well until one day, I noticed a red rash on my face, neck and chest. I felt no pain or itchiness. I tried to remember what food I ate or did the night before, but I could not come up with a reason causing the eruptions. Ben suggested that I see the doctor and I did right away. Dr. T. Purewal said that it was related to stress. Ben sent me home to rest or do some other things. I did not want to leave him but I also knew that I needed to take care of myself too, so I could keep on caring for him.

Before Ben was wheeled to the operating room, he asked me two things: To recite Psalms 23 (while in surgery and intensive care unit) and not to leave him alone while in the hospital. I promised.

# Survival . . . For Now

*"And be ye kind one to another, tenderhearted, forgiving one another,*
*even as God for Christ's sake hath forgiven you."*
—Ephesians 4:32(KJV)

I stayed in the hospital in Columbus for two weeks because of severe complications. My recovery period was not good. I barely remember any of that, only what Esther told me later.

Before my surgery, we planned in advance to communicate with hand signals in case something went wrong. Both of us had learned "deaf" hand sign language while in college and occasionally practiced it at home. This came in handy because I was unable to talk verbally when I was connected to the breathing machine (respirator).

Apparently, part of the time I was hallucinating and tried to communicate with Esther and the nurses. "I can't breathe, please, help me, I can't breathe." with hand signals, I pleaded and told Esther what to do with my chest. The nurses did not listen and kept on saying to Esther that I was having anxiety attacks.

One of my lungs collapsed and the next day the other collapsed.

I was constantly under drugs, mostly morphine. Whenever I came out from the effects of the drugs, I would try to focus on my family and turn my mind on the Lord.

Never before in my life had I prayed so hard. Although I accepted the fact that I was dying, a part of me would not give up. I pleaded with God to intervene and to do a miracle. It was a constant battle for me back and forth. Giving up and then asking God to help and then giving up. I was ready to die, but at the same time I wanted to get well. At certain times I was sure I would die any time and discouragement came over me. But then I would revive and hear myself praying for God to help. So I went back and forth for a couple of days.

After two days in the critical care unit, they moved me into a room on the Post Surgical ward. My lungs re-expanded and they pulled out the tubes. Even so, my recovery period was difficult.

I had to relearn how to eat. I no longer have an esophagus, but what replaced the esophagus was part of my stomach. It was pulled up—stretched—to my neck. I had trouble swallowing, because it takes a while before the "arrangement" replaces the function of the esophagus. I do not know about others who have gone through this, but it took more than a year before I started eating normally again.

I actually could feel the food going down into my chest. At first it was very uncomfortable. But I learned to live that way. Medically, I knew it could work indefinitely.

During the months of survival after removal of the esophagus, most people have to go in from time to time, usually about once a month, for a dilation of the scarred esophagus. Scar tissues may grow where they joined the stomach and the throat. They told me I could expect to go in for them to dilate my throat. Fortunately for me, I never had that problem.

Because I could not swallow, they tried to feed me liquid nutrients through a rubber tube in my side as well as through intravenous tubes.

It took almost two weeks before the doctors said I had improved enough to go home. Being able to leave the hospital encouraged me. Hope began to spread once again.

But my hope was short lived. After only one day, I started getting dehydrated, ran a high fever, and I was not able to eat. Esther had to admit me to Marion General Hospital where I stayed for another two weeks. While in the hospital, a portacath was inserted in my right upper chest for chemotherapy.

The hospital tried to give me things like beef and chicken broth, but Esther would not let them give me anything that was not vegetarian. I was so out of it most of the time I did not know what I ate.

Then I was home again but still with a feeding tube. I got

better and began to eat a little more each day. As my eating ability increased, so did my appetite and my strength. Along with that, my faith increased. In fact, I made so much improvement my doctor in Marion said, "In a week's time you'll be ready for chemotherapy and radiation. So you'd better eat more. Build up your resistance."

## *Esther's Reflections.....*

Ben was getting tired and weary in the hospital, so I decided to ask if he could come home and continue his care there. The hospital offered two dieticians to help me out and made sure Ben was getting enough nutrients especially protein and iron. His blood albumin was low.

I converted our dining room to a bedroom and set the bed so he could see through the window where I hung a feeding birdhouse on a tree branch to attract birds which Ben enjoyed watching when he was healthier.

Slowly, Ben re-learned how to eat and at the same time supplements like "Boost" were given through the feeding tube (jejunum tube). The dieticians advised to give him chicken and beef for his protein and to report all his daily intake.

Trying to experiment what kind of food he could tolerate was a task, but challenging. Green beans and broccoli gave him pain. Walking and at the same time back rubbing followed by hydrotherapy gave him relief.

Eager to raise his blood albumin and iron level, I tried to blend almonds with fresh garlic (to increase immune system) and gave it through the feeding tube. My children and nieces and nephews who were home felt so bad when they saw Ben with tears in his eyes and suffering severe cramping and abdominal pain after the blended food was given. With hydrotherapy and massage, he got relief and fell asleep.

My children came to visit often and sometimes my son Ben, would bring his church friends to pray for his dad. I asked Nikki one time to relieve me because I was not getting enough sleep from continuous feeding and care. She said that she was scared. While feeding Ben before midnight, I fell asleep. When I woke up, I noticed Nikki was there watching her dad. I knew she wanted to help in her own way but I don't blame her for getting scared because many times Ben needed to be suctioned to avoid choking and the feeding tube had to be flushed to prevent it from clogging.

Without meat and poultry, Ben's albumin level results came out normal.

While I tried to build up my resistance, I worked hard to learn how to change my lifestyle. If changing my way of life would help, it was worth trying.

Because my voice was not affected, I called the American Cancer Society and asked them for information. As I already knew, they said there were three options. The first was **surgery**; the second was **chemotherapy and radiation**. The third option is what they call the **alternative** treatment of cancer.

"Send me books on everything," I said, "but especially send me books on natural healing or alternative treatments."

A few days later a package of literature arrived, but I did not find anything on alternative treatments.

Thinking they had not sent everything, I called them back and thanked them for the materials and said, "But I've looked at the literature and read about surgery and chemotherapy. Where is the third kind of literature? You know, material about alternative programs?"

"I'm sorry, but we don't have any literature on that."

When I hung up, I knew I would find out.

My youngest son, Arti is wonderful with computers, and he taught me how to use the Internet. I followed every link I could to do research about my kind of cancer. I found a lot of information, but none of it was particularly helpful. The only recommendation I kept reading was chemotherapy and radiation. Everything I came up with suggested them but would not assure me that that treatment would cure me.

I stared at the screen and realized something: No conventional treatment would help. Chemotherapy and radiation were last-ditch efforts, and offered little hope.

All that week at home, I began to read the materials Esther had collected from the Adventist bookstore, as well as from friends, pastors, and church leaders. Most of them were about proper nutrition and caring for the body. She also gave me Ellen G. White's books, *The Ministry of Healing*, and her *Counsels To Health, Diets and Foods*. They're both classics in our church—written more than a hundred years ago, but still powerful, relevant, and nothing in medical science has disproved the principles she advocates. I had never actually read either of them—or if I had, I did not remember. Now as I read Mrs. White's books, I could hardly put them down.

Fortunately for me, a lot of our friends sent me books about alternative treatments. I read everything, no matter how silly the material seemed. While I read, I still kept trying to find help with conventional medicine. One of the books sent to me by friends that grabbed my attention had to do with treating various kinds of cancer without using drugs. They taught about the use of herbs as natural healers. Several books focused on eating the right kinds of foods for various types of cancers.

Esther did everything she could to get more information about alternative medicine and natural methods. She began by calling the Wellness Centers around the country and learned which ones catered to my type of cancer. We found several that worked with cancer patients, but none of them had any immediate openings. In fact, they had long waiting lists.

Despite the lack of results, I knew I was following the right path. I had already started to change my lifestyle. According to the books I read, that change of diet, exercise, right use of natural things like water, sunshine and pure air, could improve my immune system immensely.

When I left the hospital, my doctors gave me medication to prevent the acid from going into my lungs. I needed that because my stomach was right in my neck. I took the medicine for several days. The more I thought about it, the more I realized it was incompatible with the lifestyle I had now adapted. Either I was going to take medicine or I was not. It seemed to me that I had to leave it completely or take everything they offered. I prayed for guidance.

About the fourth day after I came home, I said to Esther, "I won't take the medicine anymore."

I stopped all medicine—I took nothing for the acid and absolutely nothing for pain. Even though I had undergone serious surgery, to my surprise, I never felt any pain after I stopped the medication.

Slowly, my condition improved and I started to put on weight. My doctor said, "Eat a lot, Ben, and build up your strength."

"Thank you," I said. "I am feeling stronger already."

"Good. You have a week before you begin chemo."

When I started to object, he said, "It's already late. You should have had this a month ago.

I nodded in agreement. I knew they believed the only chance for my survival was for me to have chemotherapy and radiation. For nearly two months I put off the chemo, because I had not felt strong enough. "I'm not ready," I said. "I am still too weak."

Each time my doctor spoke with me, he urged me not to delay.

Still certain I would die, I clung to God for guidance. Just knowing I was dying actually built up my faith. Strange as it may seem, I believed that the Lord could intervene at that moment or any moment. I did not think he would, and it did not matter. I belonged to God now.

In the meantime, two things happened. First was the arrival of Esther's brother, Jun. The second was information about a place that could help us.

*Esther's Reflections...*

It was very difficult to see Ben with tubes in the nose, mouth, and stomach. My youngest son, Arti, fainted when he saw his father. Then I thought of not letting my other children, Ben and Nikki, see their father in that condition. I tried to reason with them that maybe it was not best at that time. But they were crying and felt that they were strong enough to see him. So I allowed them. I do not know how I really was able to stay as strong and calm as I did. I knew it must really be God giving me all the strength I needed.

I watched Ben very carefully to make sure everything was functioning well. He slept most of the time. I kept him clean to prevent further complications. To make sure he had good circulation, I kept massaging his whole body. I kept telling myself, "I will start right now. I will do the things he can't do for himself." Sitting and trying to sleep on the chair was very hard. There were times I laid down near him so I could cuddle or hug him. The only time I went out of the room was when the children were in. That was good for me. I needed to get some fresh air, to stretch, to eat fruits and vegetables. And I was also able to cry when no one was around. The restroom became a true "rest room" for me.

I tried to make Ben laugh. Even though it hurt his incisions, he needed it. I made jokes when he complained about the tube in his nose. I tried to tickle his nose. And he complained about everything. So I just did anything he wanted me to do. At one point, he was not allowed to take anything orally and when I was moistening his mouth with a wet sponge, he bit it and did not want to let go until I pulled it out from his mouth forcefully. He checked everything too, saying the IV is not running well when it was really okay. The only time I could rest was when he'd click the morphine drip. Then he slept. But I kept watching to make sure he was still breathing. I thought about happy times. I did not want to think about anything sad. I kept his room as bright as I could. Since it was a cancer patient room, no fresh plants or flowers were allowed. I hung cards all over the walls. I did a lot of reading.

The day he was finally discharged from The James Cancer Center, he wanted to eat so badly. It was a terrible feeling that he could not swallow or tolerate food. He tried many times. I just wanted to chew or swallow for him. I did not eat most of the time when he could not. In the afternoon, he started having fever. He was restless, nothing seemed comfortable to him. I transferred him to another room of the house. I gave him medications, a sponge bath, and tried to hug him. For the first time, I felt so helpless. Nothing seemed to work. I talked to my parents and they prayed. I prayed. I wanted to have his discomfort even just for that day so he can rest. I called his doctor in Columbus, who told me to bring him back first thing on Monday. I continued to give him more sponge baths and repositioned him. I just could not keep him still. Finally I called Dr. Winegarner in Marion. He asked, "What do you think Esther?" I said, " I am taking him to the emergency room. Something is wrong." He could hardly walk. My son and I practically carried him to the van. I thank God I made the right decision to take him back to the hospital. He had pneumonia. Afraid he would choke, my son and I alternated 12 hour-shifts to watch and suction him constantly. There were times I thought, "when will all these things stop?" I did not want to give up, but at the same time I was feeling so sorry for him.

When I first went to Ohio, Jaime Pua was a partner in the practice. We had worked together professionally for almost twenty years, but our relationship never went beyond the professional level. Somewhere during those early years, the trust between us died and we never were able to become friends.

From my perspective, all the years that I was the acting chairman of the department, I tried my best to become friends with him and to build a personal relationship, but I could not seem to do that. In meetings, he sometimes accused me of showing favoritism toward others or giving myself the advantage. He often spoke up because he did not like the way I was doing things in the department. The relationship became quite strained and never improved.

While I lay in the hospital in Marion, thinking I was going to die, one of the first doctors who came to visit me was Jaime. When I looked up into his eyes, they filled with tears.

I do not think he said anything more than "Ben." But he did

something more wonderful than anything he could have said. He reached down and hugged me tightly. I hugged him back.

When we released each other, I said, "Let's forget the past."

He nodded.

I am sure he said more, but I cannot remember. I could only think of the warmth that was now between us. After twenty years, Jaime had become a special friend.

I believe that both of us had reached the point where we realized the fragility of life. Relationships, especially friendships, need to last, and for that to happen we have to put away our hurt feelings.

Just his coming to see me in the hospital was not the end of it either. Later Jaime and his family sent flowers, and I knew they were more than just flowers to a sick person. They were an expression of friendship that came from his heart.

Jaime would yet play another role in my life.

\* \* \*

I want to tell you about others who visited me. One was a doctor friend and a former partner Chuck Lui, who is Chinese. So far as I knew he had no religion. When I was lying in the hospital after my surgery, he came to my sick-bed. "Ben, I don't believe in God, and I don't believe in prayer, but this time I am going to pray for you."

He did not pray there, or at least not aloud, but I believe he did it in his own way. His last words before leaving me were, "I will pray for your healing." Those words inspired me and touched me deeply that he felt that way.

David Miller, a Urologist, came to my room after my surgery. "Now that you are sick, Ben, I feel I could easily have had your type of problem, too." He told me about his unhealthy lifestyle and the way he had kept so busy, that he had no time for anything but work. "I could be sick anytime. I think I am going to change too, because your experience makes me realize how easily I could be in your shoes." A few months later when we met again, he told me he had sold some of his real estate to spend more time with his family.

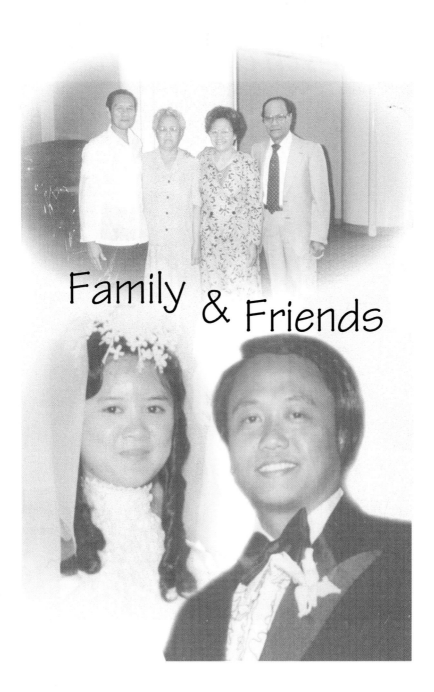

Family & Friends

# Esther & Ben

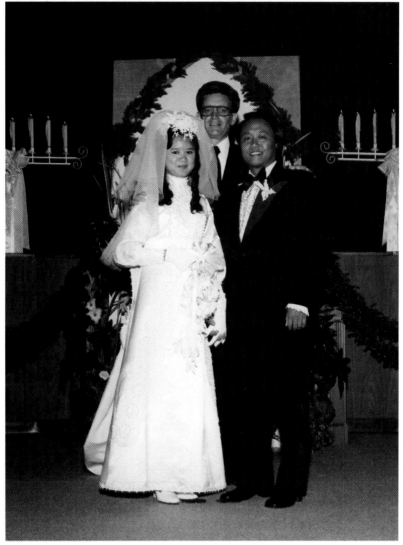

*Pastor C. Lloyd Wyman*

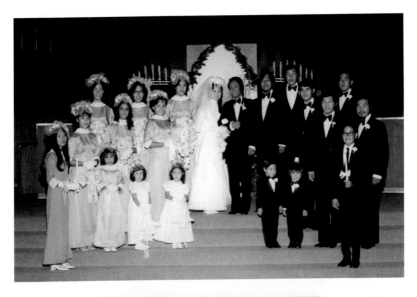

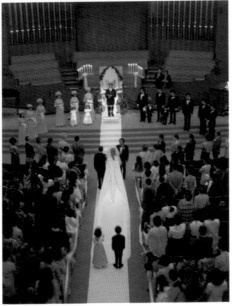

*Our wedding day, September 24, 1972 @ 6:30 P.M.*
*White Memorial Seventh-day Adventist Church*
*Los Angeles, California.*

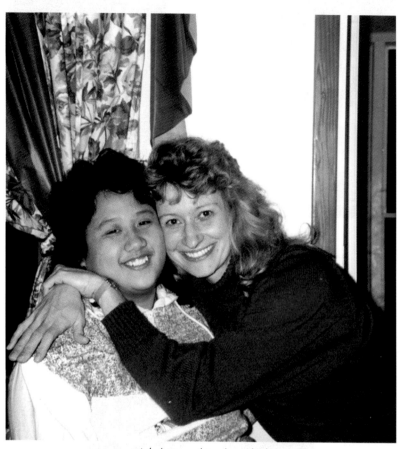

*Nicholette and Darlene Slack.*
*(Darlene received recognition for best writer . . . Associated Press.)*

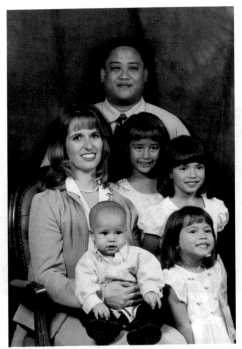

*Benjamin III, Heather, Deanna, Alexis, Kasandra, Benjamin IV*

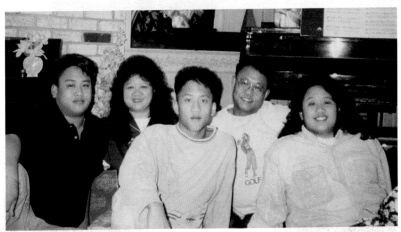

*Ore Family: Ben III, Wster, Arti, Ben & Nikki*

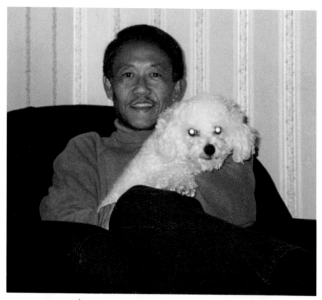

*Ben with "Prince," Faithful Friend and Companion.*

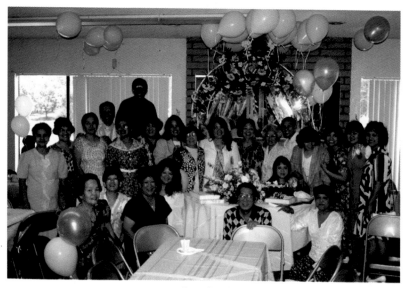

*Friends and Relatives*

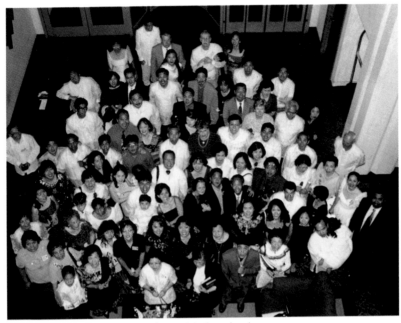

*The Sanidad-Roda Clan*

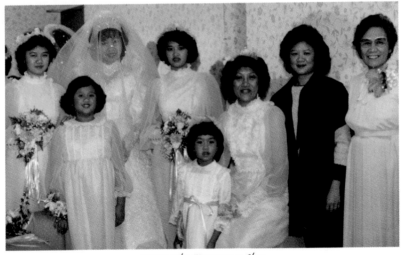

*Hernando-Tangunan Clan*

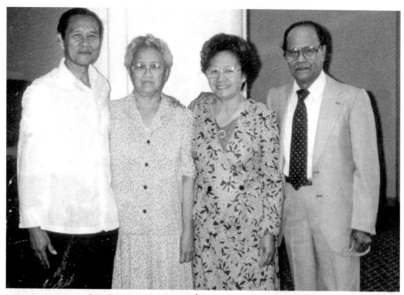

*Our Parents: Pastor and Mrs. Ignacio Hernando Sr.*
*Pastor and Mrs. Benjamin Sanidad Sr.*

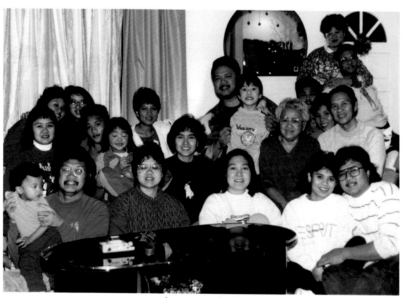

*The Hernando Clan*

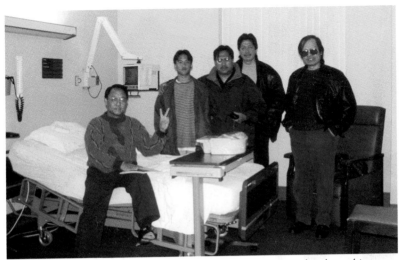

*Admission day at The Arthur James Cancer Center in Columbus, Ohio.*
*(L to R): Arti, Orly (Brother), Eddie Ravadilla &*
*Gener Romero ( Brother-in-Laws).*

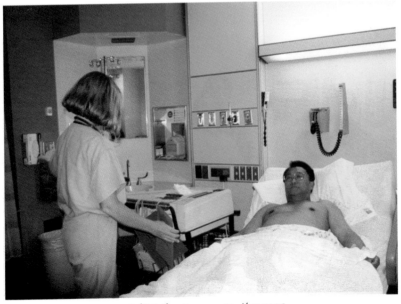

*Night Before Surgery, April 7, 1996*

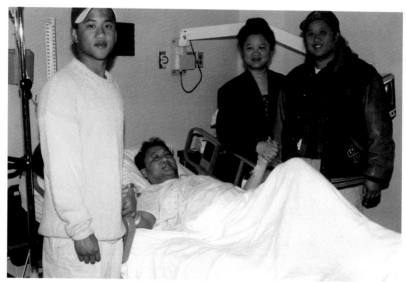

*Anxiously waiting to be transported to OR. Support from my family: Arti, Esther and Nikki*

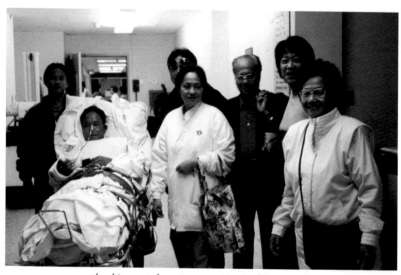

*Checking-out from Branson Hospital in Canada. Seeing me off are (L to R): Arti, Amy, Orly, Dad, Paz & Mom.*

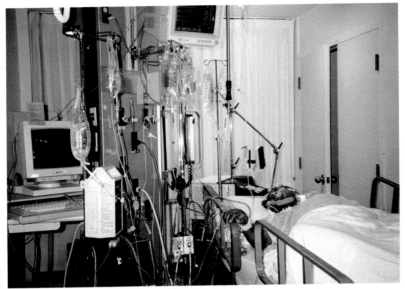

*After Surgery in ICU.*

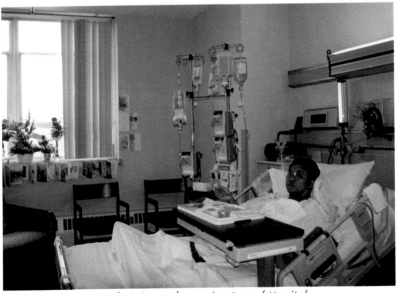

*Re-admission at the Marion General Hospital.*

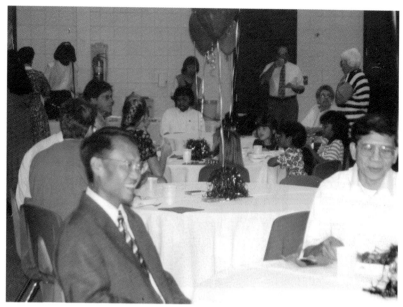

*Dr. Bayani Delos Reyes (right) and Ben.*

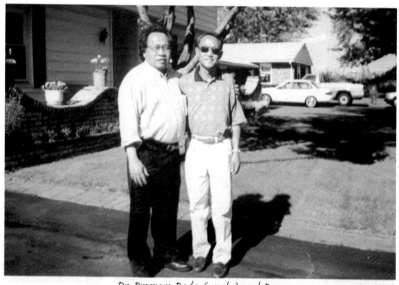

*Dr. Prospero Roda (uncle) and Ben.*

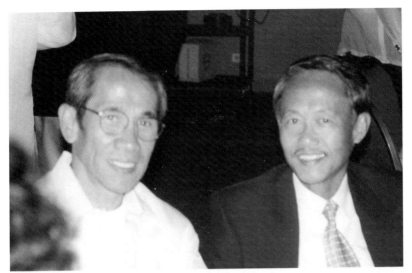

Dr. Peter Roda (uncle) and Ben.

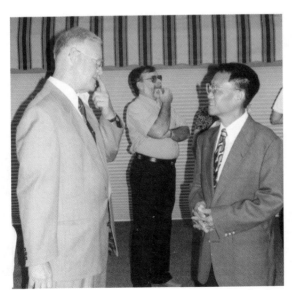

Dr. Frederick Winegarner, Ben and Mickey Holback.

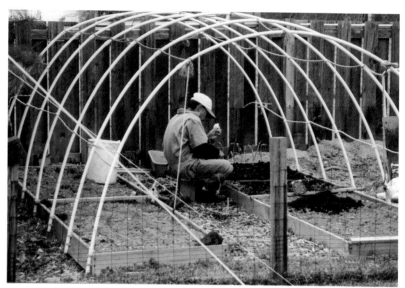

*Using organic compost made my vegetable garden
healthy which I started in July 1996.*

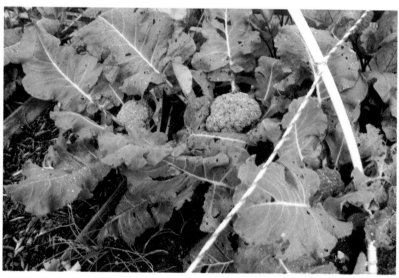

*I love "broccoli" but find it difficult to digest.*

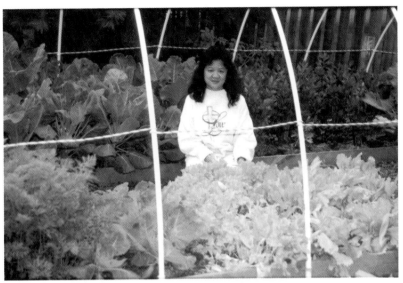

*Lettuce & carrots ready for harvesting.*

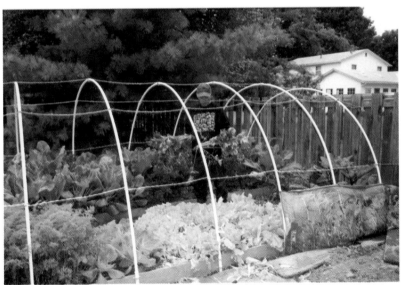

*Tomatoes, collard greens, broccoli, carrots, cabbage & lettuce in late September.*

*Participating in activities like cooking, walking, and hydrotherapy along with people who had the same needs encouraged me to change my lifestyle.*

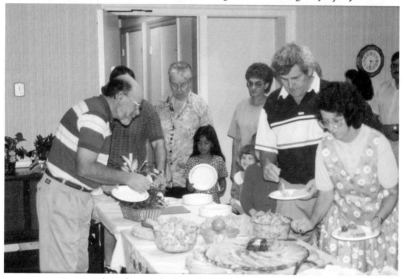

*Vegetarian meal at the Methodist Church, after cooking demonstration by Hartland Wellness Center Staff.*

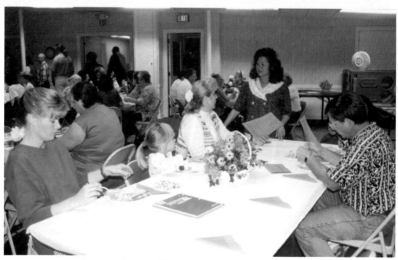

*Marion Ohio, Cooking class at the Methodist Church.*

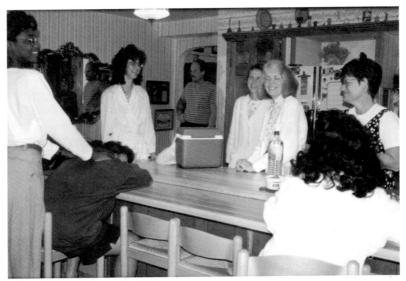

*Hartland Wellness Center Staff.*

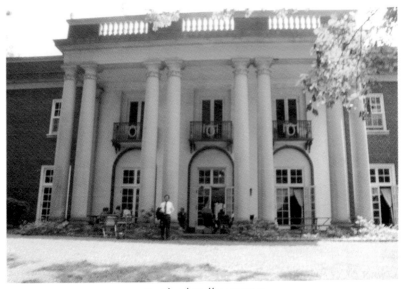

*Hartland Wellness Center*
*Rapidan, VA.*

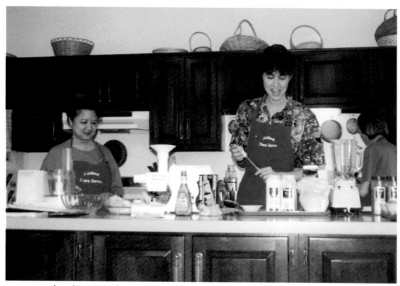

*Esther learning how to prepare vegetarian food with Juliane Aranda.*

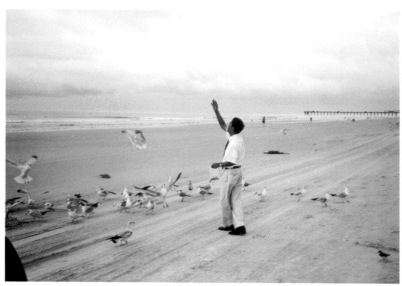

*Enjoying fresh air and the seashore.*

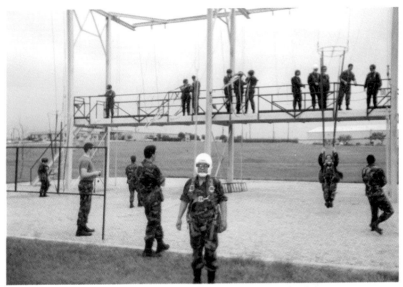

*Practicing parachute jumping at a training facility in
San Antonio Texas, Brooks Airforce Base.*

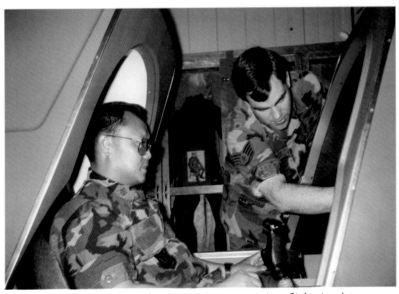

*Ben in training at Brooks Air Force Base, Texas, in a flight simulator.*

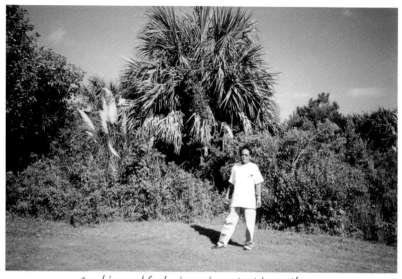

*Sunshine and fresh air are important in my therapy.*

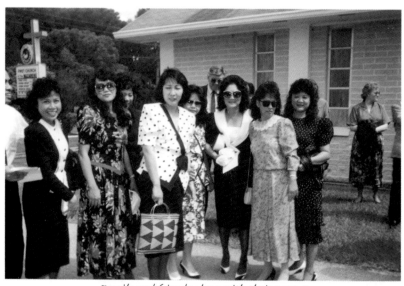

*Family and friends along with their prayers*
*brought positive effects to my recovery.*

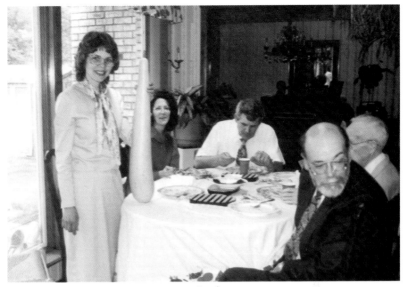

*Friends*

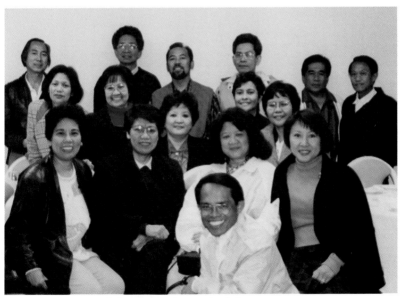

*Friends played a great role in my recovry.*

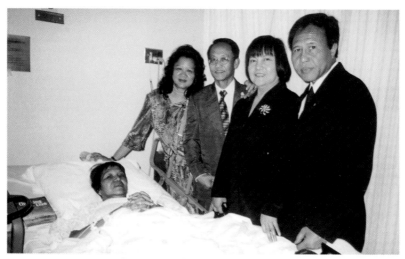

*Visiting a classmate and cancer patient with Dr. and Mrs.
Levi Pagunsan, Los Angeles California.*

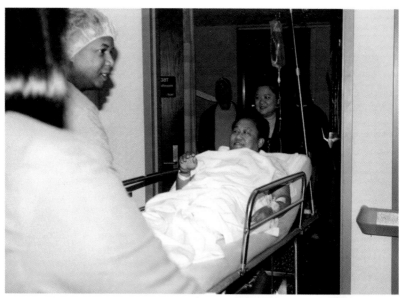

*On my way to the operating room.*

*Rainbow Express: Composed of young Christian singers from different denominations and local schools. Completed 2 recordings.*

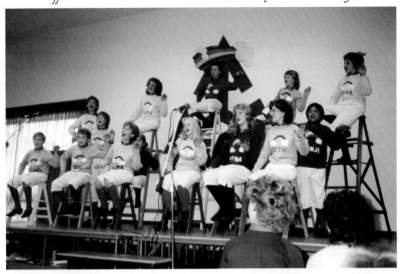

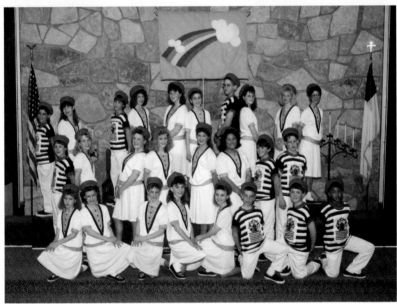

*Arti-R Nikki-second row right*

*While recuperating and unable to practice anesthesia, thank God for giving Esther, our children and me the opportunity to travel with different Christian recording artists and evangelists to help with crusades and health seminars. Traveling, meeting other people, and learning different cultures were very demanding but fun.*

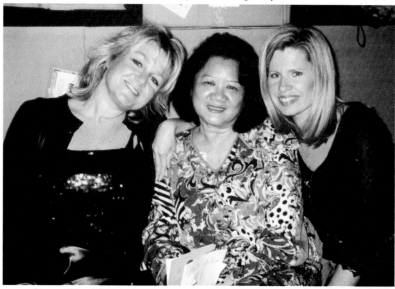

*Becki Trueblood (L) and Val Mace (R) Heritage Singers with Esther (center)*

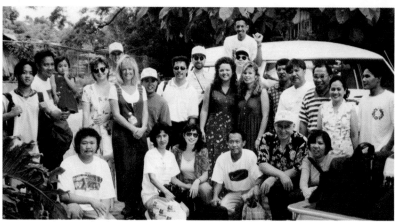

*Traveling with The Heritage Singers in their tour to the South Philippines.*

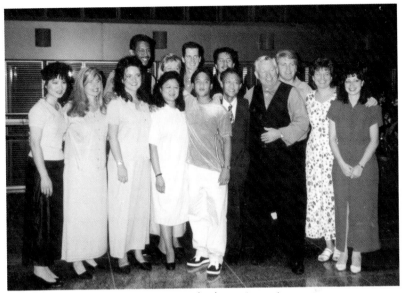

*On to Singapore with The Heritage Singers.*

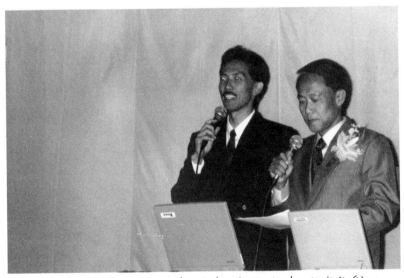

*Ben, Health Lecturer, in Medan, Indonesia. Dr. Reuben Supit (Left),*
*(Medical Director of Medan Hospital), Translator.*

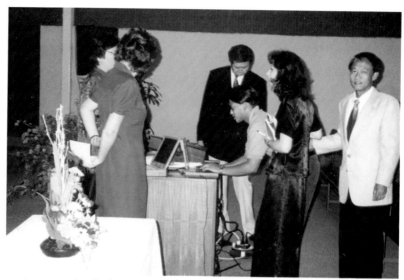

*Ben preparing for lecture in Medan, Indonesia with Dr. and Mdrs. Jonathan Kuntaraf, Jennifer La Mountain, Art working on computer and Kelly Mowrer.*

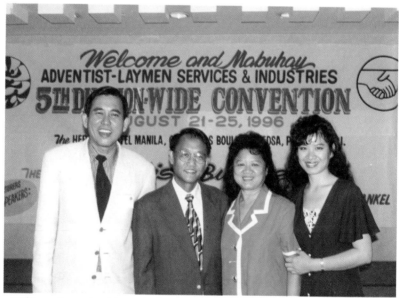

*William Cheng, President of Adventist Layman Services & Industries (ASI Asia) in Manila, Philippines, Sunshine Stahl, Christian recording artist.*

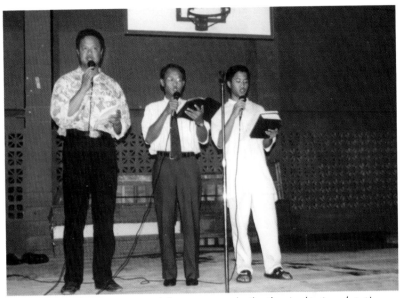

*Leading the song service with Jun Hernando (brother-in-law) and Arti, at Majuru.*

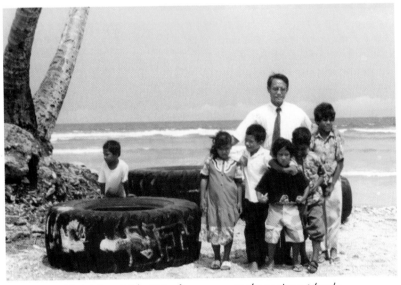

*First trip outside USA after surgery, to the Majuru Islands.*

Dr. Jonathan Kuntaraf, Sabbath School Director of the SDA General Conference Dr. Kathleen Kuntaraf (center), Health Ministries Director, of SDA General (center) watching Arti eat "Durian" fruit.

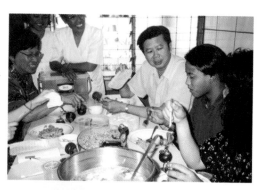

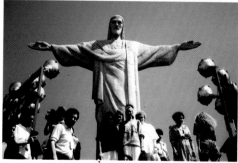

Brazil with Ullanda Innocent, Dixie Strong and Joan Rude.

Being in the midst of thousand and thousands of people accepting Christ by baptism was very emotional and awesome. Baptismal pools made of wood covered with plastic in a huge stadium in Brazil with the Voice of Prophecy crew.

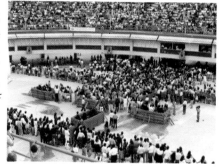

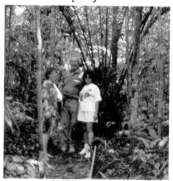

At the Amazon in Brazil, Esther hiking with Pastor HMS Richards, Jr.

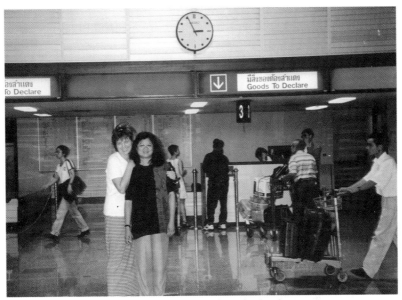

*Esther & Kelly Mowrer, at the Thailand Airport.*

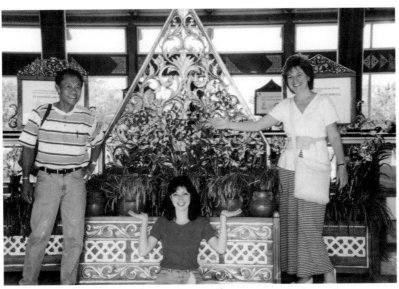

*Christian Recording Artist Jennifer La Mountain (center)
and Kelly Mowrer (right) pianist, at the Jakarta Airport.*

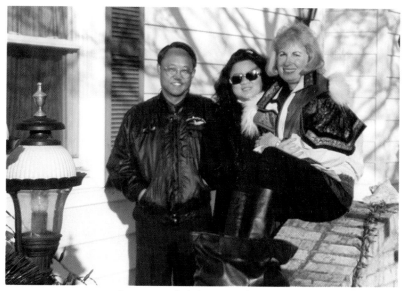

*Ysis Espana, Christian Recording Artist.*

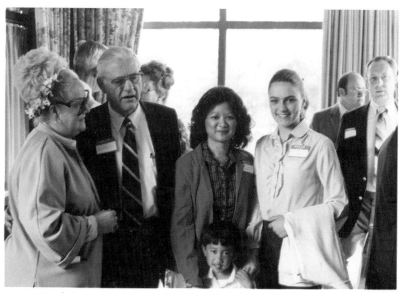

*Woody Hayes, Legendary Ohio State Football Coach (second from left),
Martha Douce (left), Esther & Arti (center), and Kristie Cook, Miss Ohio.*

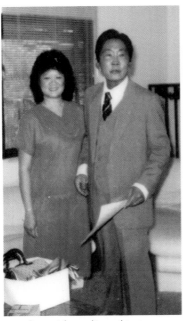

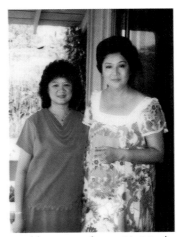

Imelda Marcos, former First Lady of the Philippines, with Esther in Hawaii.

Esther with Ferdinand E. Marcos, former Philippine President.

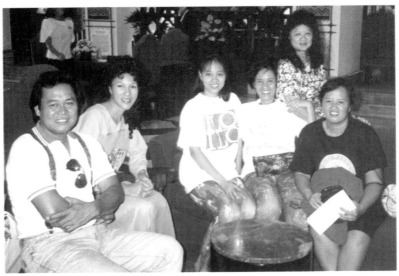

Loida Hernando with Ullanda Innocent at the Manila Plaza Hotel.

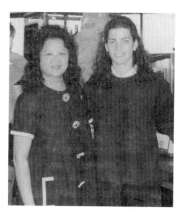

*Esther with Nancy Kerrigan*

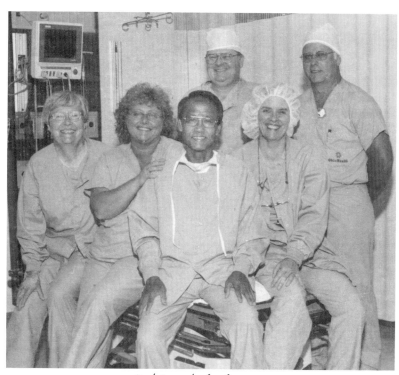

*Back to work after four years*
*Elaine Cilek, Vicki McCleland, Ben, Loretta Gamble, Jim Siverling and*
*Gary Prater, Marion General Hospital OR Staff.*

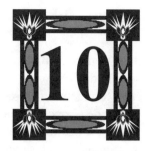

# Beyond Survival

*"My heart is sore pained within me:*
*and the terrors of death are fallen upon me."*
—Psalms 55:4 (KJV)

*"Give ear to my prayer, O God;*
*and hide not thyself from my supplication."*
—Psalms 55:1(KJV)

Many times since the spring of 1996, we have thanked God for my medical complications! The delays prevented me from starting chemotherapy treatments.

As I look back, I realize I needed time to read and to think. During that period of convalescence, I learned many things about natural health.

Esther kept me on a strict vegetarian diet, and I actually began to feel better. I was ready to set up my appointment to begin chemo when I received a letter from my aunt Elo. She enclosed literature about natural healing.

"I had cancer myself," she wrote, "and I am still alive because I followed the procedures printed in the literature. You must do as you choose, Ben. It's your decision."

She made a convincing case for me. She had chosen to turn against medical advice and follow the path I was considering.

I did not know what to do then. People on all sides of me offered advice. I read the new literature and talked to those who advised me not to have chemotherapy. My Uncle Pros, the surgeon, called me and said, "Go for everything your doctor tells you. Chemotherapy and radiation are what you need to do."

For several days I felt torn between two sides of my family. No matter where I turned, everyone seemed to know the best treatment. My wife, some of my relatives, and a number of Christian friends, said, "No, don't undergo chemo." At the same time, my parents, my brother, and some of my other relatives said, "You must go for everything medicine has to offer."

In my confusion, I knew there was only one solution: God would have to show me what to do. I prayed for guidance. None came, but I continued to ask.

As I agonized over my decision, I did not want to see in myself what I saw in my patients. I knew what death under chemotherapy and radiation looked like. If I had to die soon, I wanted to die alert and not under the control of drugs. If I have to die, I thought, I want to die naturally.

I also knew that the quality of my life would be better if I left my body alone. I might live a little *longer* with the medical treatment, but I would not live *better* and I certainly would not be healthier. If I had only a few months to live, I did not want to destroy the quality of my life in those last few months.

I had read everything I could about chemotherapy and radiation. The literature confirmed what I suspected—that they probably would not do me any lasting good anyway. At best they would give me a short reprieve and postpone death. I knew what to do. It was not any kind of flash or moment of insight, but a gradual understanding. I had the support of Esther and many friends.

"Chemo won't stop the progress of the disease," I said to Esther. "So why should I suffer needlessly? One thing more, chemotherapy kills good and healthy cells as well as bad cells."

My mind was now made up.

I pulled out the feeding tube from my side connected to my small intestines (jejunum) for nutrient feeding, out of my abdomen. "That's it," I said to Esther as I laid it aside, "I am not going to use this anymore."

She hugged me and smiled, convinced I was doing the right thing.

It took a lot of energy to make that decision. As a physician, I knew that I was acting unconventionally. In medical school, I had been taught to respect surgery and medical procedures. And now, here I was, twenty-five years later, going for an alternative treatment. Some people called it the **quack** way, but I did not care. The more I read about natural remedies and their results, the more I realized that some people were cured even though they already had lesions on their lungs and in their kidneys. They changed their lifestyle and the cancer went away. I did not know if that would happen to me, but I knew that was my only chance.

The next step was harder, so I prayed, "Lord, give me the courage to tell my doctors I will try Your way, the natural way."

With a lot of inner trembling, I made the telephone call to my doctor's office. As I had expected, he was not available so I left a message with his receptionist. Then I called the hospital and said, "I am not coming tomorrow for my chemotherapy treatment. I am canceling my treatment."

About seven the following morning, Dr. A. Chaudry, my Oncologist called. "What's going on, Ben?"

"Maybe your secretaries have told you, but even if they did not, I'm not coming over for chemotherapy."

"It's up to you, and I won't try to push you," he said. "Whatever your decision, I will support you."

I had made my decision what not to do. Now I had to decide what positive action to take.

Guidance came from a very close friend, Gayle Holback. She told Esther, "I know a place in Virginia, outside Washington, DC, that might take you. It's called the Hartland Wellness Center."

Esther called the Hartland Wellness Center, which is located in Rapidan, seventy miles south of the capital. She made the call in June, barely three months after my surgery on April 8. When she told them about my situation they said they would admit me into their eighteen-day program. They promised to send literature to explain it to us.

In the meantime, Esther had already called her brother, Jun. He is a medical doctor who also believes in using herbs and natural remedies.

Jun came with his family and they stayed with us. His first task was to teach me how to eat natural, healthy foods. He had heard about Hartland and said it had a good reputation, even though he had never been there himself. Because he knew how they functioned, he prepared me by teaching me to eat their way when I got there.

During his training, Jun had worked for a doctor who used natural remedies, so he knew a great deal about the subject. Jun cooked all our food for us. To my surprise, the food looked good, and even more surprising, it tasted good. So before I went to the program in Virginia, I had an idea how it was going to be.

The strain of the illness was finally showing on Esther, and I did not want her to get sick. I felt that if something happened to her, it would be the end of both of us.

Nikki and Arti were students at Southern University in Tennessee and just a short time before final exams they left school to be with me in the hospital. Both decided on their own that they would stay with me and help care for me—a gesture that touched me deeply. They felt it was more important for them to be with their father than to finish their school year. Even though I hated that both may have lost their college work, I believe they made the right decision. However, I felt that one of them could stay and one could go back to school. Nikki felt bad and cried when she walked to her car and drove back to school.

\* \* \*

Before they admitted me, Kae Borrero, a Hartland staff nurse, made it clear, "Dr. Sanidad, we don't look at the disease per se. Our main objective is to help you develop your immune system." Another thing she made clear was that the institution offered no false hope or miracle cures. "We don't advertise that we can cure cancer, diabetes, or anything else. We do teach you so that your body itself can heal many of your illnesses. We will build up your immune system through our program and your immune system may help you out in your diseased state," Kae added.

"That sounds like exactly what I want," I told her, and I registered.

It was not easy for us to go. Esther was caring for a woman neighbor Wilma, who had terminal obstructive pulmonary disease.

She felt she could not leave her.

"You go alone, and I will pray for you every day," Esther said. "I feel I need to be here with her." Esther was teaching Wilma to change her lifestyle and did most of the cooking for her friend. "No, you have to come with me. This needs to be a family affair," I insisted. "After I return, how will you know whether you are doing the right thing or how will you know what is the most helpful? I need you there so that both of us can learn."

Esther felt trapped, and I understood. She wanted to be with me. At the same time, she felt the neighbor needed her. If she left, she would be abandoning someone in great need. When Jun volunteered to take care Wilma, Esther felt that she had been freed to go with me. Right up until the last moment, she still struggled.

The day before we were to leave, Jun had second thoughts about taking care of the woman. "I am not so sure I can do this," he said.

"The door is open for me to go there," I said to him. "First, Esther feels she can't go and now you don't want to help."

We talked for some time and then Jun said, "Okay, I will take care of Wilma."

Perhaps part of my reason for wanting Esther was selfish, but I felt I needed her strength and her faith. I had come a long way in my relationship with God. I was growing and part of the reason was that Esther was there to talk to me and to pray with me when the doubts came. Arti came with us and later, Nikki. It would be a whole family re-education on changing lifestyle, which I recommend to every one planning to undergo such a program.

We started from Marion on a June morning and I looked forward to going to Hartland. I felt that if once I understood their program, I would get much better very rapidly.

We had driven perhaps twenty miles from home when I began to feel pain in my abdomen, a terrible stabbing pain that would not let up. Esther pulled the van into a fast food restaurant parking lot.

"I think Satan is doing something to prevent me from going to Hartland," I sighed.

We prayed and waited. After perhaps half an hour, I felt no better.

"I don't think I can go to Hartland," I told Esther. "I hurt too much."

At first, she did not know what to do, but finally she said, "If you're not able to go on, let's go back home."

Just hearing those words made me realize how much I wanted to go. I thought about all the other places not willing to take me but Hartland had said yes, about Esther's resistance, about Jun trying to back out, about Arti leaving school to be with me. So many hindrances. Yet the more difficulties we faced, the more convinced I was that God wanted us to go on to Hartland. Over and over I prayed for God to help me. If this was the right thing to do, I wanted to go.

"Let's wait a little longer," I said. While we waited I prayed hard. "Oh, God," I thought, "this is my only chance to go to Hartland. If I don't go now, I never will." I told Esther, "We'll go on. Even though I'm still in pain, we have to go. I know it's the right thing for us to do."

We pulled out of the parking lot and continued on. In a little while the pain eased considerably. In about an hour, it had gone away. The total travel took us nearly eight hours, about an hour longer than we had anticipated.

We reached Hartland just in time for the welcoming ceremonies. Everyone who had signed up for the eighteen days was already in the welcoming hall. We were the last to arrive.

The atmosphere was different from anything I had ever experienced. Even with people standing around and talking, a peaceful atmosphere filled the place. I knew we had come to a special place. For the entire eighteen days, I loved every part of the program. The people there—staff and the patients like us—were spiritual-minded, kind, and loving. Everyone seemed to care about others, nothing like any place I had been before. The facilities accommodated my family well—we could not have asked for better.

By my second day, I forgot I was going to die. A renewing process had begun and I could not remember when I had felt so well or been so happy. Just being at Hartland gave me a powerful sense of hope. Many times Esther, Arti, and I smiled at each other. We knew we were exactly where we were supposed to be.

Only a few times during those eighteen days did I think about dying. That always happened late at night when I was lying in bed in the dark and could not sleep. My mind would be alert, and then I would think about my life and the medical diagnosis. Fear would clutch at me and I would think, "I have been fooling myself. I am going to die after all. It does not matter what we do here. A few more months and then I will be gone."

Yet I did not simply accept death. For the first time, I fought it. "No, no, no," I would think, "I can't die now. I am just learning to live." Finally I would doze off and sleep.

\* \* \*

During those eighteen days I am sure the things I learned saved my life. My attitude improved. I felt—for the first time in my life—the Lord was in control. God would keep me alive as long as it pleased him.

My appetite improved and I felt myself getting stronger. At Hartland they encouraged us to walk as much as possible. The first day I tried and it was hard, and I could not even complete a fourth of a mile. The second day the walking was a little easier and I made a little more distance. Each day I walked farther. That encouraged me to push myself. At the end of the day, I'd be tired, and yet it was like an earned tiredness, and I slept better.

"I am getting stronger, healthier," I thought. "I can do things I could not do at home. I am walking and not having to lie in bed so much." Every time I did something physical and realized I could do it, I would feel a tremendous emotional lift. "I am getting healthier," I would tell Esther and Arti.

I tried to attend all the activities that were in that program—the lectures and the physical activities. I was a well-trained doctor, but as I listened, I realized how little I really knew about the body. They taught us to change our lifestyle, how to use hydrotherapy, build an exercise program. At least once a day they reminded us that we needed to get out of doors and into the sunlight every day.

Each day, we would take time and walk in the 650 acres of forested area around the institution. Often we would stroll along a river, and I could not remember any time in my life that had been more peaceful. I enjoyed the variety of wild flowers growing beside the trails, and picked some of them for Esther. I visited the organically grown vegetable gardens planted by the Wellness staff. The wild animals and birds added to the beauty of nature.

During those walks I sensed the presence of God, and my thoughts were filled with words of thanksgiving.

Of all the activities, the morning and evening worships impressed me the most. They had students at the college training to be ministers or health care givers. The Center is a part of a school where about fifty students are enrolled each year. As training for the students, they are assigned to lead out in worship and other programs like giving hydrotherapy, massage, and preparation of natural nutritional foods. Those young people studied Biblical texts and in the worship services explained them in such ways that even a child could understand. And spiritually, I was a child. I eagerly listened to everything they said.

If these children can teach me about the Bible, I thought, how much more as an older, more experienced man, could I learn so that one day the Lord can use me to help others understand? The more I thought of it, the more challenged I felt.

Just as they had promised at Hartland, my immune system was getting stronger. By the time we finished the program, I had learned a new lifestyle, my attitude was healthier, and my mind was alert.

### *Esther's Reflections...*

When I went with Ben to the hospital to get all the information and instructions for chemotherapy, I wanted to cry and tell him, "Honey please do not go for it." I felt really nervous just being at that chemo unit. While he was talking to the nurse, I walked to see other patients. They made me want to cry even more. I did not want to see him vomiting and weak. He looked weak enough. I kept talking to myself, "How can I face this one?" But I needed to be strong for him. After we left the chemo unit, I tried to keep smiling and holding his hand. He looked so confident. I had been praying, and had asked my parents to pray, that he would not take the chemo. But I had promised Ben I would support him either way. Being married to him for almost 25 years, I knew I could not argue with him. It would just make the matter worse. All I could do was pray. And I am so glad God answered my prayer. Ben cancelled the same morning. It was like a heavy load had been taken from my whole body.

# Another Threat

*"God is our refuge and strength, a very present help in trouble.*
*Therefore, will not we fear, though the earth be removed, and though*
*the mountains be carried into the midst of the sea."*
—Psalms 46:1-2 (KJV)

"Once Ben made the decision to go natural, even to leave off medication, it amazed me. I watched him do it step by step," Esther has told many people. "I have been married to him for nearly twenty-five years, but I had never thought he would make such a drastic, complete turnaround." She often giggles as she adds, "At first I was afraid he might go back, because of that drastic change. But he stood on what he believed, in what he read, and what decisions he made. I saw his strength in a way I had never seen it before. Ben had changed. And daily I thanked God for the miracle."

We returned to Ohio in the middle of July.

I knew I would live. Thoughts of death no longer troubled me. One way I showed this to everyone was that I decided to plant a garden in the backyard. It was already July when the weather in Ohio is hot and there is little rain.

"You're crazy to plant now," several of my friends laughed. "Don't you know it's too late? You won't get anything to grow now."

"We'll see," I said. I did not care about their laughter. And I did not care that much if frost came before I had produce. I had started to do something important for me—something symbolic—by showing that I believe in life.

I started from scratch—spading the soil, breaking it down, fertilizing it, and finally planting. I loved every minute I was out there working. It felt good to perspire, to know my muscles were active, and most of all that I was alive.

I did not know until later that some of our neighbors brought us tomatoes and gave them to Esther. "I'm giving these to you, Esther," one of them said, "because the doctor might be discouraged and dismayed that he won't be able to harvest his own."

To the surprise of everyone, between mid-July when I started and October when the first frost came, I produced a large variety of vegetables, including tomatoes. God had blessed.

---

### *Esther's Reflections.....*

It made me so happy when Ben decided to have a garden. It gave me more courage that he, too, wanted to be alive. Everyday I was encouraged that everything would be fine.

---

When friends and neighbors saw the change in me from a dying man to a man out working in his backyard and enjoying his life, they began to get interested in my treatment.

Since my surgery, I had lost 60 pounds, and was trim and without any fat. I looked healthy, but even more important, I felt strong and my attitude was good. Each day I began by thanking God for sparing my life.

"What did you do?" they asked. "What has made the difference?" I told them about eating vegetables, whole grains, and fruits and getting away from meat and animal products. I tried not to preach to them, because I believed their seeing me getting stronger every day was the best preaching possible, especially when all of them knew I was supposed to die within months.

Gradually my strength improved even more. I started walking, and then I took up running, alternating it with walking. Within a few weeks, I had built up my speed and endurance. Soon I was running four to five miles in an hour. Quite a difference from the man that, only months earlier, gave out after walking less than fourth of a mile.

Soon I was able to travel. For the winter of 1996, Esther and

I went to Southern California. Winter is milder and I was able to stay outdoors longer. I attended worship services in the different churches, which inspired me to listen to well-known preachers in our denomination.

One of the things we tried to do was to eat only organically grown vegetables, because too many of the supermarket variety contain pesticides and chemicals. They were easier to buy in California than in Ohio. Esther's mother and many others in the family are vegetarians. They cooked wholesome, vegetarian meals.

The weather was so nice there that I could exercise every day and get all the sunlight I needed. I became an example and living proof of total fitness through a changed lifestyle. I learned to love the fresh air, something I had gotten very little of over the years. I began to go regularly to the golf course. Some experts questioned the amount of exercise that golf provided, but it did not matter. I was in the fresh air, and that is what mattered to me.

\* \* \*

The one medical thing I have done is to continue to get checkups. Since my surgery in 1996, I have scheduled x-rays and cat scans. I always keep my appointments.

I have never been afraid of the results. Why should I? Who knows better than I do, that God has touched me?

\* \* \*

Would I ever go back to my medical practice? I asked myself that question a number of times. Each time I asked, I doubted that I would ever go back. I enjoyed my new life, although I did miss my work. I tried not to think about it, because it looked as if God had taken me out of that business forever. Unless God performed another miracle, this was now my lifestyle.

Most of all, I was happy and thankful to be alive.

Even before I got sick, Esther was involved in medical and evangelistic crusades organized by different church organizations in the US and different countries. She traveled with Christian gospel singers like **Ullanda Innocent, Pastor Walter Arties, Jennifer LaMountain, Ysis Espana, Kelly Mowrer, Sunshine Stahl, Rene**

**Pollard, The Heritage Singers** (Max Mace, director), and **The King's Herald**. And the different evangelists like, **Elder James Zachary** (Quiet hour), **Drs. Jonathan and Kathleen Kuntaraf** (General Conference), **Pastor Morris Venden, Pastor Lonnie and Jeanne Melashenko, Pastor Tim Crosby, Pastor HMS Richards Jr.** (The Voice of Prophecy), **Pastor RC Williams and Pastor Vandeman** (It is Written). We worked with the **Liwags** (Lewie and Melchor) and the **Rosetes** (Vivian and Dominador) in Florida.

"I want you to go with me," Esther said. "It's something I've always wanted—for us to do these things together."

"I'd like to go," I said, "but do you think I'm strong enough?"

"God will make you strong enough," she said.

I was getting stronger and I felt pleased that Esther wanted me to go. I wanted to be part of her work as well. Going would give me a purpose to use the life God had given back to me. I chose to travel with her and have never regretted. Now instead of going back to work, I had found another way to practice medicine and use my talents.

In the Marshall Islands and the other places we have been, we worked closely with evangelists. They preached about Jesus Christ. Then we offered them physical help. We felt it was a complete program for the whole person.

I found great joy in doing simple medical procedures.

At night before the evangelists preached, I gave short lectures about using natural remedies that I had learned at Hartland in the program they called **NEWSTART** (see Chapter 14). When I lectured, I shared my own experience with them along with the information I had learned. I could say, "I know this is true and that it works, because it saved my life."

I loved the travel to the Far East with Esther's projects. From there we visited Indonesia, Thailand, India, Singapore and the Philippines. At each of those places, I was able also to share my experiences.

It was a ministry. Now I was truly living a life for others. I was exactly where God wanted me.

* * *

We returned to the U.S. on October 3. After a few days of rest and catching up on everything, Esther and I decided to drive to Toronto and visit my parents. We had not seen them since my surgery.

On October 9, Esther and I, our two-year-old grand daughter, Deanna, and our dog Prince got into our van and started to drive. We were having a fine time, listening to tapes, singing, praying, and praising God for the wonderful time we now had together. As we drove along, I thought, I feel stronger and healthier than I can remember. It is wonderful to be alive!

Then it occurred to me suddenly; I remembered a dream I had the night before. It was so real that it woke me up in the middle of the night shaking.

"I saw myself lying on the operating table with my belly open," I told Esther. "What does this mean?" "Is God telling me something?" I added.

"I, too, had a dream," She answered, "and I was working in the intensive care unit caring for a patient."

"Why these dreams? Will I have surgery again?" I sighed.

Nothing did warn us, none, except our dreams that night on what would happen next, a few hours later.

\* \* \*

Just about the time we reached the outskirts of Toronto, a sharp pain struck my abdomen, like a sharp knife cutting into me. At first, it was like sharp gas pains, but they worsened. They felt almost as if someone was tightening a screw around my upper abdomen.

"Something's wrong," I said to Esther as I clutched my abdomen and groaned from the pain. If anything, my suffering worsened. No matter how much I forced myself to relax or how much we prayed, I got no relief.

Then came the nausea and vomiting.

"We're going to a hospital," Esther said.

I moaned in agony. Right then I did not care what we did. I just wanted relief.

As the pain continued and did not let up, my mind went into panic. "The cancer has returned," I thought. "All this time, I've been in the Far East talking about diet and nutrition and how healthy I was. And now it returned. I've been kidding myself."

Then I thought of how good God had been to me. Before my surgery, I had asked God to give me six months. Later I learned that Esther had asked God to give me a year. Almost two years had passed and I was alive. I had already beaten the statistics for my type of cancer.

Yes, God had given both of us more than we asked for. As I thought about dying, I did not want to die, of course, but this time I was not afraid. "I'm ready to go home to you, Lord Jesus," I whispered through clenched teeth. "If that is what you want, I am ready."

Maybe it sounds strange; I was scared that I would die in a foreign country. I kept thinking, I want to go back to the US and die there. I thought that probably all the months previously, even though I had done my checkups, my cancer had been growing, and suddenly it obstructed my bowels. But I was not as scared as I had been when I originally developed the cancer.

Esther brought me to the emergency room at Toronto's Branson Hospital when a problem came about. "Who will take care of Deanna and Prince?" Esther thought frantically.

Suddenly, a tall, composed woman appeared. Esther beckoned to her. She came right away and said, "Go get help and I will watch them for you."

"Are you a Seventh-day Adventist?" Esther asked instinctively. She answered, "Just for you, I am right now." That did it. Esther ran to the ER while the lady talked to me in a soft comforting voice. She took care of our grandchild and called my parents afterwards while Esther was with me in the ER. We learned later that the lady was there to see a friend and we believe the Lord sent her at the right time and right place to help us!

While we waited, my suffering did not lessen. They injected a painkiller, but it did not help. They took x-rays and did blood tests. Finally, I fell asleep, mostly from exhaustion and the effect of the painkillers.

My parents came to the hospital. After we had been there perhaps two hours, my sister Amy, who was a nurse there, arrived. She heard me scream with severe pain and was so frustrated that nobody had alleviated my suffering.

Apparently she saw a doctor she knew well, who was walking down the hall on his way to the surgical department to operate. "Please, please come to the emergency room and look at my brother," she begged.

He came in to see me and examined me. Then he said to her, "Your brother needs an operation. It's an emergency."

I did not hear any of that, only what Esther and my sister told me later. Esther did say that the surgeon had to rush up to his scheduled surgery because his patient was already on the table. Another two more hours lapsed before the same doctor got back to me.

As I remember, I waited in the emergency room between six and seven hours before they took me into surgery. During that time my blood pressure fluctuated badly—way up and then it would dip dangerously low. The last time I heard it before they wheeled me away, the systolic pressure was in the low 80s (*the top figure that needs to be at least 100 to be considered normal*).

As they put me on the gurney, I stretched out my hand and Esther took it. Despite the agonizing pain, I stared into her eyes and I saw her love for me. "Sweetheart, I think this is it," I whispered, "I'm going to die." I said good-bye, believing I would not come out of the operating room alive.

"No, you are not going to die. We will see to it that you survive."

Esther had a strong faith, but I hurt with too much pain to believe.

I did not know what had happened. I was kept sedated most of the time. According to Esther, after the doctor operated on me, he came out and told her that he discovered that my intestines were already dead and black.

Apparently I had had an obstruction in my abdomen, which had been caused by the scar tissue that had developed between the wall of my abdomen and the intestines, where the feeding tube was removed. The intestines twisted around the scar tissue causing an obstruction of my bowel, which then prevented the flow of blood to more than half of my intestines.

"I've removed the obstruction and there's a possibility—the very slightest possibility—that blood would flow again through the intestines," he said.

"Can't you do anything else for him?" Esther asked.

He shook his head. "I can't do anything except watch." He explained that he was not sure what part to resect (*cut*)." He told her he had packed the bowel with a hot towel. "The hot towel may help return the flow of blood to the intestines. Now we wait and see if anything happens."

A short time later, the doctor came out. "It's good," he said. "It's good, the intestines have started to come alive again!"

In that short time—less than half an hour—the bowel had started to change color, to "pink up." After the surgeon had released the obstruction, my bowel started to move.

He could not close my abdominal incision, because I had hemorrhaged inside the intestines, which had bloated because of blood. He had to drain the intestines. At the same time he transfused blood. He gave me a total of seven units of blood.

Less than an hour later, the surgeon and the anesthesiologist came out and said, "It's a miracle; it's a miracle."

The following day the surgeon operated on me again to see if the intestines were still alive.

On the fourth day the surgeon became concerned that he did not hear any bowel sounds and I had started to develop a fever. That meant that my intestines were not functioning. He planned to operate on me again the third time to see if he had missed anything.

"That is enough," Esther said over their objections because she believed that I had already undergone too much pain and suffering. She decided instead to bring me back to the USA where I could get better medical care.

She chartered an airplane ambulance and transported me back to Marion, Ohio. My doctors did not operate on me but gave supportive care and treatment such as intravenous protein.

For five days after surgery, I did not know what was happening. I thought I was unconscious. But Esther said that I had been talking a lot. My children thought that I had brain damage because I could not remember any of them and I sounded incoherent and confused.

After two days in Marion, I started to recognize the friendly and smiling faces of the doctors and nurses at Marion General Hospital.

"Oh, so I am alive, again," I said to my family. It felt so wonderful to know I was alive. I recovered quickly.

On November 15, five weeks after my surgery, we went back to Toronto to visit my parents as we had planned before. On that trip, I wanted to stop by Branson hospital to thank the surgeon. I was not able to see Dr. Feinberg personally, but I spoke to him by phone. I also met the nurses who had taken care of me. I thanked all of them profusely.

Finally, I was able to spend a few days with my parents. My mom and dad hugged me tightly and were very happy I had survived once again.

## *Esther's Reflections...*

I wanted Ben's parents to see that their son was doing great. So we decided to drive to Canada, without knowing we would soon experience another nightmare. This time it was worse than the cancer surgery. As we drove, we listened to music, trying to recall all the goodness that God gave us everyday. Then suddenly Ben felt an intense pain. In my whole life with him, I never saw him with that kind of pain.

Many times he asked me, "Can I scream?" I told him to scream as loud as he could. He was really in so much pain. Then I saw his stomach getting distended. I was still trying to be calm. I was so helpless, wanting to hold him but I was driving. I could only pray. And I kept telling my granddaughter, Deanna, who was two years old, to keep praying for Grandpa. Then she told me, "But I already did, and grandpa is still doing it." (screaming with pain).

After we had found a hospital, and Ben was taken to surgery, I waited, knowing that if the doctor came out later, that was a good sign. But if he came out in a few minutes, that would mean he could do nothing to help Ben. The doctor came out in a few minutes.

It was a very tough decision to make whether to take Ben back to Ohio or to let him stay in Canada where he was with his parents and siblings. But I thought about his wonderful care and support in Marion the first time he was sick. And I was not able to rest well in Canada. I needed to stay strong for him. My children helped me realize that he was mine now, and only I could make the decision. He was not fit to fly because of his condition. Either way I was taking a risk.

I frequented the restroom. Just the word "restroom" made me feel good and rested, even without a real rest. I used that place every time I needed to talk to the Lord. Inside the restroom I could turn on the faucet to hear the water flow and it made me think of a refreshing waterfall. I thought about trees, red roses, birds and yellow butterflies. I sang many times, "It is well with my soul."

When I came out of the restroom, I knew that Ben and I needed to go back home in Ohio.

The "angel" who came to help at the ER was Glory Gage, a Canadian recording artist.

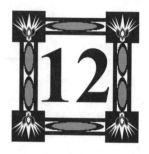

# Understanding

*"And as it is written, there is none righteous, no, not one; There is none that understandeth, there is none that seeketh under God."*
—Romans 3:10-11 (KJV)

After our chartered plane arrived at Marion from Toronto, I needed to have a line put in the vein in my neck. This is called an intracath—a tube to feed me intravenously. It's an invasive procedure, that is, it's more than sticking a needle into one of the peripheral veins, because they have to do the procedure in the operating room.

Jaime, my former colleague, was on call. If our relationship had remained strained, I would probably have refused his services. And knowing Jaime, quite likely he would have refused me as a patient. The strain between us was gone. We were friends and I offered myself under his service.

He tried to put the needle catheter into my neck. He did not succeed because my veins were collapsed.

Esther said that he came out of the operating room and talked to her.

"I am very sorry, so sorry I couldn't put in the intracath."

"It's all right," she said. "Ben will understand."

Shortly after that, Dr. Winegarner inserted a line through the subclavian vein on my left upper chest. That took care of the problem.

---

### Esther's Reflections...

Jaime came out from the OR to explain to me his difficulty in inserting the intracath. I was not bothered about his unsuccessful attempt. He tried his best and showed his sincerity. I was happy that after 20 years of strained relationship Ben and Jaime finally reconciled.

Another anesthesiologist colleague, Dr. Rhee, came to my room after that procedure, and we talked for a few minutes about our families. We had not known each other really well, but it had been a relationship of mutual respect. As we talked, I gathered that, in many ways, he was a man like me. He worked many long, extra hours, which meant he did not spend much time with his family. "You know, Ben, I may not even know my children right now," he said.

"Then you need to change," I said.

"Yes, I know that."

"Don't wait or put it off," I said. "I am blessed to have a second chance, but you might not. We have to show love to our family in spite of how busy we are with our work. What happens if you keep on working and then you die? Will it be worth it?"

"Yes, I can see from your experience how short our life is," he said reflectively. "One day it looks as if we will live forever, and then something like this happens."

"That's right. So don't wait. Enjoy your life now. Enjoy your family," I said.

"I am going to change my lifestyle. I'm going to get closer to my family."

He meant that. The next week, he started going to church with his family, which he had not done often before.

Such experiences have helped me understand how God works in our lives. People sometimes learn more about God from the way we handle problems and life-threatening illnesses than they do from the positive things we say and do.

Not only was I thankful to be alive, but also so grateful that God could use my life and my illness to touch other lives.

# A New Life

*"Then shall thy light break forth as the morning, and thine health
shall spring forth speedily: and thy righteousness shall go before
thee; the glory of the Lord shall be thy reward."*
—Isaiah 58:8 (KJV)

In 1996, I began to make radical changes in my life. Because
I was a doctor, I read everything I could find about the conventional
methods of treating esophageal cancer.

As I expected, they offered me no help. It forced me to realize
that the one and only Great Healer is God. With God's help and my
wife's support, I made drastic changes in living a healthy lifestyle.
And they worked!

Some people who read this might think, "Oh, I see, Ben went
into remission." Such things do happen; but it did not happen to me.
This section of the book is not about **remission**; it is about a **cure**.
Remission means the body, for unknown reasons, stops producing
cancer cells. The term also means it may reoccur as quickly as it left.
In my case, my immune system slowly killed the cancer in my body
and freed me.

I began with surrender. "God, you have control over the remaining days of my life." I prayed that way many times and meant it. "If it
is your will, you will prolong my life so I may continue to have a more
productive life to serve You and others."

I was at the end of my life. For me, there were no other options.
First, I had to get rid of the bad, unhealthy habits I had accumulated
in my lifetime. They included: overeating, drinking alcohol and caffeine; eating the wrong kinds of foods; living a sedentary life without

exercise; staying indoors and doing less outdoors; frequenting polluted areas; being immoderate or intemperate in my activities; staying up late at night; overworking for twenty years; uncaring about my body or my mind; allowing stress even on trivial things.

Despite my commitment, I still had trouble and felt frustrated with so many things I had to change, but with God's help, I kept on.

Within a remarkably short time, I had cleaned up my diet, which was the biggest struggle in my life. I not only learned to eat healthful food, but I learned to enjoy it immensely. I stopped eating meat and highly processed foods. Studies show us that beef, pork, fish, chicken, and turkey are "biological reservoirs" of parasites and a source of infection.

Once I learned that fact, I adopted an important rule: As much as possible, I would eat chemical-free food. Sick people like me can not afford to let our immune systems fight other infections while the cancer cells grow. And once started, they tend to grow rapidly.

From then on, I was a vegetarian. Plants are at the bottom of the food chain and less likely to carry parasites and chemicals to the body. The more natural the food, the safer the diet.

On the plus side, fruits and vegetables are "body cleaners" and not only aid our digestion, but assist in the elimination of waste. The most important factor in fresh vegetables and fruits, however, are the hundreds of vitamins and minerals they contain that strengthen the immune system and fight many diseases, including cancer.

When we had returned from our eighteen days at Hartland, Jun my brother-in-law, cleaned out our refrigerators and threw away all the unhealthy things we had been eating.

He replaced them with fresh fruits, vegetables, whole grains, and nuts.

Immediately some people said, "No meat of any kind? That's fine, Ben, but what will you do without protein because you don't eat meat?"

"Not a problem," I tell them, "Instead of meat, I eat nuts, whole grains, and soy products such as tofu. Research shows that most vegetables contain a few of the amino acids that make up protein. If we eat widely, we never have to worry about not getting enough protein."

In all the months since my illness, protein deficiency has not been a problem!

The Seventh-day Adventist church has long held to the principle that God's original diet did not include meat. They point out that the human race never ate meat until after the flood, and God allowed meat eating only as an accommodation to the human race.

For many years, people looked on Adventists as odd and their diet as strange. In the past twenty years, that attitude has largely disappeared. Others are now accepting the lifestyle that our church has proclaimed for a century and a half. A number of athletes, politicians, and entertainers have become stringent vegetarians. Their open advocacy has caused an increased interest in a vegetarian lifestyle. Consequently, many vegetarian restaurants have now sprung up that prepare tasty, healthy food. Today, most traditional restaurants offer vegetarian entrees. My friend, Cecil Murphy, who is the president of a writers' organization has monthly dinner meetings. In advance, they ask for "regular" or "vegetarian" meals. Also, if you order in advance, most airlines will serve vegetarian meals.

* * *

Once I went chemical free, my next step was to stop drinking carbonated and highly sugared drinks. I replaced them with fruit juice, herbal tea, and vegetable juice. As I learned, juices contain flavonoids that strengthen the immune system. For the first time in my life, I began to drink large amounts of pure, uncontaminated water. And I have learned to love it.

After that, we did a thorough house cleaning. We threw out anything that contained chemicals such as benzene, lead, and arsenic—poisons that are found as supposedly harmless ingredients of many solutions. Once inside the body, those chemicals destroy the cells and, in turn, they cause malignancies such as breast and prostate cancers.

I also learned a great deal at Hartland about mental hygiene, this is based on the premise that the body and the mind interact and that much of the illness of the body springs from illness of the mind. Ancients knew what we're just beginning to accept: much of our body's ill health is functional rather than organic.

Now euphemistically referred to as "psychosomatic medicine," the problem has become pervasive in our stress-filled society and our physicians and hospitals are still not adequately addressing it. Although this is changing, they are still too prone to look at curing symptoms rather than eliminating the cause.

Physical therapy was our next step. The premise on which this therapy rests is that the body itself is the only healing agency and physical therapy helps the body fight disease. This does not suggest using physical therapy as an exclusive means to treat patients, but rather using an appropriately balanced program between the use of drug therapy, surgery, and physical therapy in the treatment of disease. This makes a radical change. We are saying that treatment is for the patient rather than aimed at the disease.

In the following pages, I offer you my understanding of what I have learned since my change of lifestyle in 1996. Most of the information came during my stay at Hartland Wellness Center.

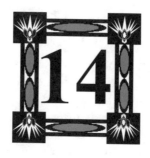

# God's Way

*"Pure air, sunlight, abstemiousness, rest, exercise, proper diet, the use of water, trust in divine power—these are the true remedies. Every person should have a knowledge of nature's remedial agencies and how to apply them. It is essential both to understand the principles involved in the treatment of the sick and to have a practical training that will enable one rightly to use this knowledge."*
—Counsels on Health, page 90

After numerous phone calls to healing and wellness centers, God had led us to the Hartland Wellness Center in Rapidan, Virginia, where I learned to apply their eight natural remedies to health. I went there for a total lifestyle change, which included my commitment to follow their teachings. And I changed.

I liked the fact that they kept things simple. They based all their teachings on eight simple principles, using the acronym **NEW START.** That makes it easy to remember and apply their methods. And best of all, as far as I was concerned, they based everything on the use of natural remedies.

Those natural remedies became the basis of my healing. They are all simple and available to everybody because they come from nature. I want to explain these eight natural remedies. It is because of them—and the grace of God—that I am alive today.

## EIGHT (8) important factors of Health

| | | |
|---|---|---|
| N | = | Nutrition |
| E | = | Exercise |
| W | = | Water |
| S | = | Sunshine |
| T | = | Temperance (or moderation) |
| A | = | Air |
| R | = | Rest |
| T | = | Trust in God |

## N Stands for NUTRITION

For the first fifty years of my life, I ate anything I wanted and seldom thought about health or nutrition—fast foods, dairy products, meat—it did not matter. If I wanted it, I ate it.

My first lesson to accept in Natural Remedies was the emphasis on eating fresh fruits, vegetables, whole grains and nuts. Again and again, they reminded us that the less the food is processed, the more fit it is for the human body. Processing food destroys some of the vitamins and minerals. "The closer to nature, the better," is something I must have heard every day at Hartland. Another saying I liked was, "The shorter the distance from the garden to the mouth, the better."

Here are some of the other things I learned about nutrition:

### 1. Our bodies were created to eat fruits and vegetables, not meat.

One of the surprising things for me to learn—and I smile when I think that I practiced medicine for twenty-five years and did not know this—is that our teeth are meant to chew fruits, vegetables, grains, and nuts. They are not made to tear flesh food the way animals do. When we compare human teeth to that of animals such as dogs, tigers, lions, monkeys, or wolves, they all have canine teeth—made to chew meat.

Their digestive tract is short. When they eat meat, they digest and eliminate it quickly, within a few hours. We humans, however, have longer digestive tracts. It normally takes healthy people about 24 hours to digest and eliminate fruits and vegetables. When we eat animal or flesh food, studies have proved that those foods often stay inside our bodies 48 hours or longer with many people. That delayed elimination causes constipation.

As most people now know, vegetables, fruits, and whole grains contain a lot of fiber, and fiber is essential in the elimination process. This means that when we eat a diet without meat products, we eliminate fecal matter in about half the time. When I was a big meat eater, I suffered regularly from constipation. Since I have turned to a wholesome, vegetarian diet, I am no longer constipated.

When flesh foods stay in the body a long time, they can become carcinogenic. An immense amount of research has shown that heavy meat eaters run a high risk of cancer in the intestinal tracts. For such people, the meat stays there and rots inside the tract. When the body finally absorbs the chemicals or toxins that are produced when the meat rots, it can then cause cancer.

Of course, not every meat eater will get cancer, but they face a greater risk. "Why take the risk?" I asked myself. I wanted to do everything I could to be as healthy as possible.

Since my surgery in April 1996, I have not eaten fish, poultry, or meat. I am a vegetarian, or what they call lacto-ovo vegetarian. That is, I eat limited amounts of animal products such as eggs, milk, cottage cheese, or cheese. Others, who call themselves vegans, eat no animal products

I changed my lifestyle by avoiding flesh foods. It is important for me to say that I did not think of it as giving up anything. Sometimes people act as if I have gone on some kind of diet where I give up the things I like to eat. For me, it was a choice—a choice for health.

Even now, people will say to me, "What can you eat?"

"I can eat anything," I tell them. "I choose not to eat a lot of things."

## 2. We need fat—the right kind of fat.

Studies now indicate that the more animal fat people eat, the higher their levels of cancer risks.

The ideal diet is to eat fat as it occurs naturally in vegetables, whole grains, and nuts. Vegetable fats contain no cholesterol, and they do not carry the viruses such as salmonella or mad-cow disease that are carried by living creatures.

I have a friend who grew up in a home where they fried almost everything, and most of it in animal fat. He did not like food that was raw, boiled, steamed, or baked, and especially he did not like vegetables. After he married a woman who did little frying, he agreed to eat anything she put on his plate. Within weeks, he had turned away from fried foods. "When I went to my parents' home and ate," he said, "sometimes I left with heartburn."

### 3. We need to avoid fermented food, such as vinegar.

If apple juice is exposed too long to the air, it ferments and is changed to alcohol. If there was anything hard for me to give up it was Tabasco sauce. I have always loved spicy foods and sauces. Even when I ate fruit, I added Tabasco sauce—something I learned to do when I was in the Air Force. I did it because the food was so bland and there was always a lot of Tabasco sauce around.

Along with this, I now teach people to eat small amounts of (or avoid) food that is pickled, smoked or salt-cured. I urge them also to avoid alcohol. Despite occasional news of health benefits, the risks of using alcohol include cancer of the liver, mouth, pharynx, larynx, and yes, the esophagus.

### 4. We can use herbs to enrich nutrition.

For instance, we can use herbs, dried or fresh, instead of salt to enhance flavor. Low-fat cooking methods often require more seasoning to keep food flavorful. Herbs can satisfy that need without adding calories.

Here are 10 common herbs that most people can grow in small gardens or pots or indoors, and have them for flavoring throughout the year.

• Basil: Best when used fresh, because it loses most of its flavor when it is dried. It greatly enhances the taste of tomato sauce, pâtés, creamy sauces, and pesto. Basil is also good on fresh or cooked vegetables.

- Chives. More gentle than onions, we can use chives in soups, sauces, and salads. I like to sprinkle it on baked potatoes.
- Dill. Although best known for its use in making pickles, it can flavor sauces and salads and potatoes. It is best to use fresh, because dill loses its scent when dried. One suggestion for dill is to use it with chives, garlic, parsley, and yogurt for a low-fat dip or topping.
- Mint. One of the most popular herbs, mint can garnish or flavor drinks, soups, sauces, salads, and fruit desserts. It is good fresh or dried.
- Oregano. This herb is widely used in Greek and Mexican dishes as well as a seasoning for pizza. Oregano enhances salads. It is usually better dried.
- Parsley. Use parsley as a garnish and flavoring for sauces and soups. Sprinkle it on potatoes or vegetables.
- Rosemary. Because it is quite pungent, use rosemary sparingly. If rosemary is picked before it flowers, then dried and crumbled, it keeps well; fresh, it can be bitter.
- Sage. Good in tomato soups; dried sage is preferred over fresh sage.
- French tarragon. The fresh is superior to dried and only the leaves are edible and can be used to flavor mushroom recipes, and in creamy soups and sauces
- Thyme. Use it to flavor soups and sauces. Commonly used in French food, especially in cream sauces. It keeps well dried and may taste less bitter than when used fresh.

**5. We can not neglect fiber.**

Almost everyone today knows the benefits of fiber, or at least they know they need more fiber in their diet. At Hartland I learned that by eating fiber-rich food, I could eat a larger volume than just meat products. The fiber-rich diet is that which is found in beans, nuts, vegetables, fruit, and whole grain products such as bread or cereal. Ground flax seed, a good source of fiber also lowers cholesterol by absorbing cholesterol in the intestines. It also contains linolenic acid, which is claimed as anti cancer.

Fiber forces us to chew more, takes longer to digest, and

because such foods stay in our stomach longer, makes us stay satisfied longer. Then fiber speeds food through the large intestine. (*For those who want to lose weight, more fiber can result in a more rapid weight loss*).

**6. Our need for protein has been greatly exaggerated, especially by the dairy industry.**

First, most vegetables have a small amount of protein. If we eat a wide variety of foods, it is almost impossible not to get enough protein.

Excessive consumption of protein places a heavy burden on the body, especially the kidneys. Many nutrition experts used to say the body needs about 56 grams of protein a day—that figure is now seriously in question. More recent studies indicate that the body's need is about half of that amount. Even so, 56 grams of protein is equivalent to a three-ounce beefsteak. Or, as I learned, half a cup of roasted soybeans, sunflower seeds, or peanuts provide the same amount.

\* \* \*

Within the past few years, pharmaceutical companies including Warner-Lambert, and Whitehall-Robins have entered the herbal supplement business. Bayer alone planned to spend twenty-five million dollars in 1998 in promoting its herbal line of products.

Here are the major herbal products the pharmaceutical companies are marketing:

*St. John's wort* to treat modern depression.
*Kava kava* to fight moderate anxiety.
*Black cohosh* to relieve symptoms of menopause.
*Saw palmetto* for the treatment of moderate, benign prostatic hyperplasia (BPH).
*Valerian* for the treatment of insomnia.
*Echinacea* to prevent and treat colds, flu, and boost the immune system.
*Ginko* for age-related cognitive decline.
*Horse chestnut seed* to promote leg circulation and to protect against leg swelling.

159

*Ginseng* to boost mental and physical resistance to stress.
*Garlic* to lower mildly elevated cholesterol and tryglycerides.

## E is for EXERCISE

Exercise is very good for the human body. Most people know that today. For example, people who are physically active tend to weigh less, have lower blood pressure and serum cholesterol levels, and as a result are at a much lower risk for heart disease than their inactive counterparts.

Research studies indicate that Harvard University alumni who exercised regularly could expect to live 2.2 years longer than their inactive counterparts, and that the improvement in longevity could come from walking or jogging eight to ten miles a week. (*New England Journal of Medicine 314 [1986]; 605-613.*)

As an ancient proverb says, "Every man has two doctors: his right leg and his left."

Consider the benefits:

Exercise:
- Increases blood circulation because the exercised muscles massage the blood vessels.
- Increases HDL (the good cholesterol) that removes and eliminates bad cholesterol from the body and helps to prevent atherosclerosis.
- Helps to control the appetite and thus control weight.
- Improves the digestion and enhances the regularity of the bowels.
- Provides mental refreshment, by drawing blood away from the congested brain to neglected muscles.
- Decreases anxiety, depression, and mental stress.
- Increases a general sense of well being, short-term ability to think, and enhances the self-image.

For me, exercise means moderate amounts and not the kind that overtaxes the body. When I began to exercise, I realized I needed to choose an exercise that I enjoyed. Some people enjoy exercise machines, but I find them boring.

No matter what form we choose, we need to do it in moderation. Too much exercise stresses the body. Too many live with the idea that if a little is good, more is better. It's better if we think in terms of "What is right for me?"

Those who exercise regularly are more in tune with their bodies. They know when to cut down or when to keep going.

* * *

"Walking makes for a long life," a Hindu proverb says.

More health experts are advocating walking as the best source of exercise for most people. As someone said, "Walking is cheap (*all you need is a good pair of shoes*), you can do it almost anywhere at any time, and you can do it alone or with others. Walking uses all of the body's 206 bones and 660 muscles.

Take care of your feet. Buy shoes that are comfortable and large enough for each toe to be free. Make sure they are lightweight and flexible. Good running shoes with well-cushioned heels and insoles work fine. I suggest you buy them late in the day when your feet are the largest. When you walk, wear thick, or double-layer socks that help wick away perspiration and prevent blisters. Most athletic stores carry such socks.

Here are helpful ideas on walking:

- Stretch. Before we walk, we should stretch our muscles and our joints in order to avoid injury in our tissues when we walk. Now when we grow older, our flexibility becomes limited. So if we do exercises every day, it will help us in our flexibility and our balance. Not only that, when we exercise outside especially, it invigorates the body muscles and increases the circulation in muscles and makes our stamina stronger.
- Start slowly. If you are beginning, do not overdo it. Walk up to five days a week and slowly build your distance and endurance. The first week, for example, you may choose to walk 10 minutes a day and then go to 15 or 20 the following week. For most people, a 45-minute walk, at least five times a week is usually enough.

- Walk habitually. We are starting on a new lifestyle. Think of it as a lifelong habit.
- Walk correctly. Good posture fosters good respiration and blood circulation. It also prevents or reduces back strain. Stand tall, look ahead (not at your feet) and swing your arms. If you want to walk faster, bend your elbows to a 90-degree angle and make an arc from the waist to the chest with your hands.
- Walk faster. Take quicker steps, not longer ones. If you walk about four miles in an hour, that pace gives your cardiovascular system a good workout.
- Walk up hills. Choose places to walk that give you more strenuous exercise. When going up inclines, lean forward slightly to ease the strain on your leg muscles; when going downhill; take shorter steps to take the stress off your knees.
- Find excuses to walk. Find ways to fit in extra steps throughout the day. One friend uses the stairs at any building whenever he goes up five or less flights. At the mall, he parks his car a long distance from the stores. Even when using an escalator, he walks rather than standing still.
- Pick the right time of day—for you. Someone suggested to me, "Keep that commitment to exercise as if it were an important business appointment," and added, "Think of it as business—healthy business."
- Walk for yourself. I like to remind myself and others, "I am not in competition with anyone. I don't have to push myself beyond my level of comfort. I need to exercise enough to enjoy my health, not enough to overtax my body."

Although some health addicts still chant, "No pain, no gain," we are now learning that it does not work that way. Moderately vigorous exercise suits the body best, which is one reason many are turning to walking. Good, regular exercise not only strengthens the heart and slows it, but helps us to stay younger longer. It can help our whole circulation become nicely balanced. Most fitness experts suggest that we exercise at least three times a week, but every day is even better.

A twenty-year study published in the JAMA tracked the death

rates of nearly 16,000 Finnish adult identical and fraternal twins. They concluded that regular exercise can help extend the life span of every individual, regardless of genetic makeup.

They asked the twins, among other things, about their ongoing level of physical activity and used that information to put them into one of three categories: (1) Conditioning Exercisers. Those who reported exercising for at least 30 minutes six times a month. (2) Occasional Exercisers exercised very little; and (3) Sedentary those reported no regular exercise.

Their research indicated that the Conditioning Exercisers reduced their risk of death by an average of 43 percent when compared with sedentary types. Even Occasional Exercisers reduced their mortality risk by 29 percent compared to non-exercisers. It reminds me of a saying that goes, "If you can't find time to exercise, you will find time to be sick."

## W is for WATER

The body is about 60 percent water and the brain is about 85 percent. That is about 40 quarts for an average person.

The water is inside cells, around cells, and even in our bones. Our body uses 40,000 glasses of water each day to take nutrients to each cell as well as carry away waste products. Our body has been designed to recycle almost all of that. However, we do lose some of it each day—which we need to replace.

There are three best times to drink water:

• Between meals
• Half an hour before a meal
• Two hours after a meal.

Those who know the most about nutrition suggest that we not drink with our meals because water dilutes the digestive juices and it slows down our digestion.

By getting adequate amounts of water each day—48 to 64 ounces—most Americans could alleviate one of the most prevalent health concerns in our country: irregularity. Americans spend around

200 million dollars a year on laxatives. A better and less expensive way is to drink enough water.

By itself, water is not a laxative, but when combined with a high-fiber diet, it bulks up the stool so that the stool, becoming soft, can go through more rapidly.

There are two ways to use water. The body uses it internally. These days, most people who care about their health understand the need to drink eight, eight-ounce glasses, or a total of 64 ounces of water each day. If we are doing intense, physical work and perspiring a lot, we need to drink even more.

Many people do not realize the need to replenish their water the first thing upon arising. At night we lose two or three glasses of water just by our respiration. Just about the first thing I do when I get up is drink two full glasses of water. That amount replaces what I lost at night. I usually drink water and regulate it during the day until I get at least 64 ounces.

Someone has said, "A drink of water is like taking an internal shower. It rinses your stomach and prepares it for work. It helps you overcome sleepiness and the temptation to snack between meals."

"Why so much water?" someone asked. "Why aren't two or three glasses enough?"

That was a good question. And there are a number of reasons:

- Water eliminates our body's chemicals and toxins and the products of metabolism.
- Water is used in the production of saliva and hormones,
- The digestive tract needs water for mixing various digesting juices with our food and for transporting nutrients throughout our body
- Water aids in the digestion of food.
- Water also helps in the battle for weight loss because it dilutes the waste products when fat is broken down inside our bodies.
- When used externally, water cleanses the body and the pores in the skin.
- Water helps to excrete impurities and wastes from our body through sweat on the skin and urine through the kidneys

- All cells in our body need water.
- We could not even use the oxygen we breathe unless our lungs were moistened. We could not swallow, blink or even speak without water. Even our brain needs water to function properly.
- Blood cells float in serum, which is largely water.
- Water helps regulate our body temperature.
- When water is combined with heat (hydrotherapy) and body massage, it helps strengthen the immune system.

\* \* \*

"I drink whenever I am thirsty," I have heard people say. Thirst, however, is not a good indicator of our water needs. Typically, most people only replace about two-thirds of the water they lose because they do not feel thirsty. Our bodies are such that we don't feel thirst until we lose one percent of our body's total water supply.

People who don't habitually drink water may need to force themselves at first. Make it a habit. One man I know starts with two, 10-ounce glasses in the morning, and while he works, he makes certain he drinks at least another four full glasses. He likes to keep water at his desk and sip throughout the day.

The warning most people need is that it is water they need and not just liquid. Typically, they take in between two and four cups of water through their food. Although the body uses water in any form, sugared drinks have calories that are digested like food. Cola contains phosphorus that depletes the body's supply of calcium and contributes to osteoporosis (*brittle bones*). Chemicals in diet drinks include flavorings, preservatives, and colors that irritate the stomach lining. Black coffee and tea force the liver and kidneys to detoxify and dispose of them—a process that demands extra water.

\* \* \*

Too many people confuse thirst with hunger. So they nibble instead of sip. Recently I said to an overweight man, "The next time you feel hungry between meals, why not sip an 8-ounce glass of juicy, no-calorie-filled water?"

He raised an eyebrow and I said, "If there's not enough flavor, why not a slice of lemon, a squirt of Real Lemon, or rub mint across the rim of the glass?"

The one complaint we often hear is that if we drink at least 64 ounces of water, it guarantees that we will visit the restrooms often. "If I drink all that water, I will have to run to the toilet ten times a day!" "So what's wrong with that?" I ask. "Consider the benefits. It also forces you to do a little more physical activity, especially if you have to go up and down stairs."

\* \* \*

Finally, I urge people to consider hydrotherapy, something else we discovered at Hartland.

In hydrotherapy we increase the temperature of the water and subject our bodies to it for 30-45 minutes.

We need to have a hydrotherapy tub. Some people go to the spa, but usually the temperature is not high enough. We need a temperature of at least 103 degrees. Most spas have temperatures about 100.

I think the old-fashioned steam baths or a whirlpool works all right.

The point of hydrotherapy is that it opens the pores of our skin and releases our bodies' toxins when we perspire.

At Hartland, I think I used it just about every day because I was ill. They monitored my core temperature, and when it reached 102-103 degrees Fahrenheit, they maintained that temperature for thirty to forty-five minutes. After the treatment, they poured cold water over me to close the opened pores.

The rationale is to create an artificial fever every day. When we do that, we produce more white blood cells—the kind that fights infections. When we have many white blood cells in circulation, it increases our immune system. That, in turn, makes us healthier.

### S means SUNSHINE

We need sunshine, in moderate amount—30 to 50 minutes a day before ten in the morning or after three in the afternoon.

More than getting a nice tan to help us look healthier, the sunshine offers immense benefits to us. Most of us take the sun for granted and use it more as a marker between day and night than anything else. Yet the sun has many health-giving properties—and it is free. Here are some of those benefits:

- It provides vitamin D that our body needs. When that vitamin is lacking, calcium absorption is deficient and bones become soft. This results in rickets in children and osteomalacia in adults.
- It brings out our natural oils (cholesterol) in the skin. Sunshine lowers the level of blood cholesterol.
- It is an excellent sterilizing agent. The sun's ultraviolet rays destroy bacteria.
- Most of us would be amazed at how beneficial sunlight can be in the treatment of infectious diseases; it improves energy and fitness, lowers our blood pressure, decreases our resting heart rate, increases the storage of glycogen (*sugar*) in the liver, which then lowers sugar levels in the blood,
- Sunshine strengthens the immune system and increases our body's tolerance for stress.
- The rays of the sun enhance the beauty of the skin.
- Research now indicates that when we are exposed to sunlight, it prevents depression and it enhances our mood.

Before my cancer, I worked inside the operating room all day. I seldom went outside into the fresh air and sunshine. It was often dark when I went to the hospital and I seldom returned home before the sun set.

Although there were other factors involved, I now know that lack of sunshine contributed to my feeling tired and grouchy. I also know that since I have made it a daily practice to get a lot of sunshine, I feel better and my mood is lighter.

Unfortunately, a lot of people think negatively of sunlight because of the high incidence of skin cancer. Some of that comes about because of over-exposure to the sun's rays, with the old theory that if a little is good, a lot is better. But another factor is the amount of fat in most people's diet.

According to Dale and Cathy Martin, fat…creates a basis for the formation of free radicals…which are molecules that are very unstable and can damage every system in the body. Exposure to excessive sunlight intensifies the activity of these rabble-rousers to the point that a deranged cell can have its genetic order scrambled and begin to act like someone gone mad.

Experiments have been done where a group of rats was put on a very low-fat diet…and another group of rats was put on a high-fat diet, similar to what most Americans eat. What they found was that it is very difficult to produce skin cancer in the rats that were on a low-fat diet, whereas the rats that were on the high-fat diet readily produced skin cancer.

So while 450,000 people are diagnosed as having skin cancer every year, most of this cancer is in the form of a benign basal-cell or squamous-cell cancer, precipitated by excessive sunburn, high fat diets, and low levels of vitamins C, A, E, and selenium, which are found primarily in foods of plant origin. These three vitamins and mineral function as guardians of the cell, among other things, playing a major role in preventing the radicals from doing any damage. *(Dale & Cathy Martin, "Living Well" p.123, as quoted by Jeff and Marlene Wehr, "Taking the First Step," vol 1, No. 1, p6).*

* * *

**What about skin cancer?** True, sunlight is the major risk factor in skin cancer. Most of the 40,000 new annual skin cancer cases in the United States could be prevented if people would protect themselves against **over-exposure** to sunlight.

Most skin cancers are readily curable. The most serious and rapidly growing is malignant melanoma, and it accounts for 75 percent of the 7,400 skin cancer deaths each year. Following breast cancer, it is the leading cause of cancer in women. Especially vulnerable are those ages twenty-five to twenty-nine.

The U.S. National Cancer Institute predicts that one of every six Americans will develop some form of skin cancer. Skin pigment melanin protects us by filtering some of the ultraviolet light that comes through your skin. This explains why light-skinned people have more skin cancer than those with darker skins. If you are blond, you are more susceptible than brunettes. If you are African-American, you have the most melanin in your skin and the lowest incidence of skin cancer.

For those of us who enjoy exposing ourselves to the sun, here is a good principle to bear in mind: **Shorter, multiple exposures are better than one lengthy exposure.**

We need to concentrate on a general revitalizing of our entire body. However, if we must be exposed to the sun for long periods of time, we can help ourselves by wearing protective clothing and putting sunscreen lotion on unprotected skin areas. However, if we want to get the most benefit from the sun, we would not use sunscreens, oils, or lotions because they inhibit the oil-secreting glands of our body from working properly.

We also need to get the sun directly on our bodies—outside— and not from inside our house. Glass filters out up to 95 percent of the beneficial ultraviolet rays.

So let us enjoy the sunshine and think of it as a special gift from our Creator God.

### T refers to TEMPERANCE

Temperance means to avoid the things that are bad for the body and mind, and to use the things that are good in moderation. Unfortunately, we even use some of the good things to excess.

One of the most important things to eliminate for me was caffeine. I drank it to excess. Research says moderate amounts probably do not hurt. I think, however, it is wiser to eliminate it altogether because caffeine is an addictive substance.

I suggest we avoid all alcoholic drinks. Some of the experts point that alcohol, when taken in moderation, is good for the circulation. But I would rather not touch it when I can find better ways to help me physically. What they often do not point out is that we can get the same beneficial effects from grape juice! And juice does not hold the potential for addiction or the cause of serious problems.

Cigarette smoking has to be right at the top, along with caffeine and alcohol, I tried that as well. In fact, the three of them seem to go together.

For me, smoking was more a social thing, and I never liked it that much or became addicted. But about one-quarter of the population is addicted. More and more evidence points out that we also need to be free from secondary smoke. Too many have developed emphysema and other respiratory ailments just from being around those who do smoke.

There are a lot of small things we use that most people probably do not even think about. Vinegar is one, which I've mentioned under nutrition. I used to love to pour vinegar into my rice. That meant too much fermented food and too much spice. I tried to moderate them, but always went back. After my surgery I was able to cut such things down to almost zero.

Here is a brief overview of the importance of moderation in several areas.

**Food.** A little fat is good, but the American diet of 30-40 percent fat produces tremendous complications for our body. The same holds true for salt and sugar.

Although you need a variety of food, it is better to eat fewer foods at a meal than a large variety that introduces unnecessary complexities to the digestive process. Research also shows that you are wise to avoid unhealthy combinations such as milk, sugar, and eggs.

Six to seven cans of diet soda a day will erode tooth enamel because of citric and phosphoric acids, commonly used as flavor enhancers. Although we need about 64 ounces of water a day, if we take in that much plus the same amount of diet soda, we can overwhelm our kidney's ability to excrete the liquid. It could result in symptoms of nausea, lightheadedness, and possibly even seizures.

**Rest and sleep.** Most of us need seven or eight hours of sleep, and that does not seem to change, as we get older. Unfortunately, we live in a society of sleep-deprived people. Some of them even boast that they get by with four or five hours of sleep a night. They may be getting by—for a while—but one day their body will rebel. One way it rebels is for something to go wrong. We call that getting sick.

**Exercise.** Regular exercisers frequently outlive competitive athletes. In addition, people who constantly push their bodies in training for competitive sports frequently put stress on joints that results in permanent cartilage damage.

**Work** is where we probably need to look most for moderation. Think of it this way: When we overwork, it means neglecting something else, usually our family. And I know that from my own experience. When cancer struck, I realized that the trade was not worthwhile.

In short, we need to avoid extremes of any kind. I have a friend who barely survived a heart attack three years ago. He has become so health conscious that he is now an extremist, almost as bad that way as he was with his prior lifestyle. He is terribly correct in his eating habits, but he is not very pleasant to be around. At a mutual friend's house, he lectured the hostess about the rich, sugary dessert she served. He could easily have said, "No, thanks," and let it go. But for the next quarter-hour he subjected all of us to a lecture on the dangers of a bad diet.

Before closing this chapter, I want to offer a few suggestions on how to live temperately.

Make gradual changes. In my case, I had to make drastic changes because it was a matter of life and death. But that is not true for most situations.

Set small, easily obtainable goals. We need to be careful not to try to change everything at one time. It is better for us to start out by walking one-fourth of a mile and gradually building up than it is to try five miles the first day.

Temperance means moderation. It does not mean stress. If we have to push ourselves to do more, we are probably overexerting ourselves.

Consider the values of temperance: It helps preserve our health, enables us to maintain our energy level, gives us a sense of having control over our desires, and brings balance into our lives.

### A is for AIR

For most of the twenty years I worked in the hospital, I did not breathe pure air. I stayed in a situation where I breathed recycled, operating room air—and they are not the same.

I learned the importance of pure air—by that, I mean outdoor air. Air that is purified. Especially when you are at the seashore, the beach, and a flowing river or in the forest, we all know that the plants absorb the carbon dioxide and clean the air. Then out comes pure oxygen, and we breathe pure air.

Because we are aerobic creatures, we need fresh air to sustain life. Every day we take more than 17,000 breaths to keep our body fueled. Human beings can live for weeks without food and days without water, but only minutes without air. Without the oxygen in the air, we cannot carry on the minimal activity needed for survival. For most people, six to eight minutes without oxygen causes irreversible brain damage.

Air is one of the things our bodies require to live. When we breathe—and I had to learn the right way to breathe—we enhance our health because when we breathe correctly, we eliminate a lot of carbon dioxide and toxins from our circulation.

One of the things they taught us at Hartland was to open curtains and lift up the windows to let the air come in. Even at night, the fresh air from the outside is good for us to breathe. In fact, it is even more important because at night the air is less polluted. We only need to crack our windowpane a little, and then make sure we are not exposed to a draft.

People are finally getting concerned about the quality of air we breathe. And we need to be. Even nonsmokers who live in high air-pollution areas suffer with the same kinds of symptoms that smokers do.

The pollution in the air decreases the amount of oxygen that can actually get into our blood streams. A prevalent ingredient in polluted air, carbon monoxide, actually binds with the oxygen in the blood, making it ineffective. In fact, according to at least one study, tens of thousands are dying every year from the effects of air pollution.

According to an article in the December 9, 1996, issue of *Time:* "Major cities in the United States kill thousands of Americans every year, but not by crime or traffic accidents. The victims' only mistake is that they breathe: if people live and breathe long enough in city smog, they usually contract some disease that will eventually kill them."

**How we breathe.** Part of our life quality depends on the way we inhale and exhale.

Most people use less than half their lung capacity in breathing. Shallow, improper breathing reduces vitality and causes the metabolic rate to slow down. That then brings on tiredness. It affects memory, creativity, and concentration, as well as judgment and willpower. It is really quite simple. If we use our abdominal muscle and habitually inhale and exhale deeper, we can decrease such symptoms.

We also know that breathing affects the way we feel—something of which many people are unaware. Or to say it another way, strong emotional feelings affect our breathing. When we are angry, afraid, or nervous, we tend to take shallow, rapid breaths.

Tension alters our normal breathing patterns. Fear increases tension and tension restricts breathing, which shows the intimate relationship between body and mind. We know now that suppression of emotion results in muscle tension that limits respiration.

Most people know that when we breathe deeply and slowly, it calms us. That is why we hear people say things such as, "Take a deep breath." Or "Breathe deeply and count to ten before you speak." Those are calming methods. If we calm ourselves when excited, nervous, angry, or worried, we feel more relaxed, more positive, and even have a stronger sense of self-esteem.

By contrast, we know that those diagnosed, as schizophrenics tend to breathe with the upper chest diaphragmatic breathing. To help them move toward a normal life, many therapists just teach such patients to breathe properly.

Here are tips to help us breathe better:

- Exercise outside. It is better to do this in the mornings when the air is cleanest.
- Wear loose-fitting clothing. Tight clothes tend to constrict breathing.
- Breathe deeply—which comes with practice.
- We need to concentrate on breathing from our diaphragm—down at the bottom of our lungs.
- Spend as much time as possible among trees. Pine trees seem especially good for lungs.

\* \* \*

Despite all we have learned about pollution, we still take in too much contaminated air. Among the pollutants we breathe in are carbon monoxide, sulfur oxide, sulfates, nitrogen oxide, benzopyrene, ozone, cadmium, and mercury. This contamination comes not only from industrial waste and auto emissions, but also from tobacco smoke. (*Of course, polluted air is better than no air.*)

Tobacco smoke, as mentioned earlier, is the most common indoor pollutant. In the Live-Longer Lifestyle studies, we could not compare smokers with nonsmokers because we have such a small number of smokers among SDAs. However, we did have a fairly sizable segment of members who had previously smoked, so we gathered data by following them and their lifestyle.

When we compared nonsmokers to former smokers (*those who had quit for at least a year*) it surprised us to learn that their **longevity** was about **the same.** Individuals who had quit before the onset of disease were able to reverse and even regain most of what they gave up in health losses due to smoking. There is, however, a point beyond which to stop smoking would not help undo the damage. Once we develop such diseases as lung cancer, emphysema, or other cancer-related diseases, it is too late.

Research now indicates some surprising results from breathing polluted air and has shown we can reverse these symptoms when we breathe pure air. Some of them are: drowsiness, depression, fatigue, nausea, dizziness, headaches, cardiovascular disease, cancer, leukemia, skin rashes, irritation of eyes, ears, nose, lungs, and sinuses.

### R means REST

When they spoke of rest at Hartland, they meant more than sleep. We need to rest or cease from eating. Too often, people eat a heavy meal just before going to sleep—and I used to be one of them. That means we do not give our digestive system a chance to rest. That part of our bodies must work while the rest of the body tries to rest. It does not work very efficiently.

Then almost as soon as we awaken in the morning, we eat breakfast. This means our digestive systems never get a good rest and must work continuously.

We need to rest our stomach. One way to do that is to eat a small amount of food at night, such as fruit, which is easily digested. We ought to have at least three hours of non-eating before going to sleep at night. If we do, then our digestive systems can rest with our whole body.

Someone once said, "God gave us the day to work and the night time to rest." I have learned the value of that statement. Sleep is important, far more important that most people acknowledge.

At a conference, a speaker once said, "We have so many things going on you'll have to miss a lot of sleep to take in everything. But sleep isn't that important anyway, is it?"

The audience responded with loud clapping.

Sleep is more than important—it is vital to good health. Here is the most significant fact for us to bear in mind: During sleep our **bodies regenerate** themselves. As the breathing slows and deepens, nerves and muscles relax and we produce less heat. When the digestive system rest, the cells of the body can rebuild and recuperate, and prepare us for the next day.

Research says that most people need seven to eight hours of sleep every night. It also points out that those who sleep less tend to live shorter lives. Much study is now going on in what is called sleep deprivation. Those who regularly sleep less than five hours or more than ten should see their personal-care physician. Spending too long or not long enough time in bed are both unhealthy.

At night, most of us experience 4-5 cycles of sleep of about 90 minutes' duration. We begin with light-to-moderate levels of sleep in cycles 1 and 2 and they last about half an hour. Slowly our bodies move into cycles 3 and 4. They can last anywhere from 10 minutes or as long as 30. Then we drift into the fifth cycle, which lasts 10 to 30 minutes. In that deepest level we do most of our vigorous dreaming. Stages 3 to 5 are where the healing and rejuvenation take place. Our bodies diffuse stress and anxiety, and we move into a more peaceful, deeper quality of sleep.

This means that we need not only the right quantity of sleep—7 to 8 hours—but the right quality as well.

Here are things we can do to make our rest more meaningful and beneficial:

- Vigorous exercise during the day in the fresh air aids in restful sleep.

- Have an abundant supply of fresh air in the bedroom when we sleep.
- A nighttime routine that may include a warm bath, reading, drinking herbal tea.
- Avoiding stimulating activities such as exercise, TV, or negative conversations.
- Avoid heavy eating at night. And especially, do not snack before bedtime.
- Avoid drinking beverages containing alcohol and caffeine.
- Set regular hours for sleeping.
- Make it a rule of "early to bed, early to rise." Because of the circadian rhythm, which is regulated by the sun's rays, the deepest sleep occurs between 9 p.m. and midnight.

The principle I want to emphasize is simple: **We need to sleep well to stay well.** Yet millions of people still don't know that or else they consciously violate it by their sleep-deprived lives. Estimates say that as many as 30 percent of fatal crashes come from drivers who fall asleep at the wheel. In the United States, at least one in every twenty people has caused an accident by nodding off while driving. Most such accidents occur between midnight and 6:00 a.m. It is not the long drives, the late hours, the boredom of expressways, or the lack of light. It is an unwillingness to admit the need of sleep because of a hyperactive lifestyle.

Too many of us shave hours off our sleep to work longer, spend more time with the family, do household chores, play golf, or chat on the Internet.

That means, sleep is not a high priority. Worse, many people have been sleepy for so long they do not know what it's like to feel wide awake. Chances are that every one of those sleep-deprived people is less than fully alert and their performance at work or school shows.

Many blame sleep deprivation on our 24-hour society where electric lights, 24-hour businesses, TV sets, and electronic highways encourage us to put off going to sleep. We must depend on alarm clocks to get us going the next morning. To make it worse, many sleep-deprived people brag about their less-than-adequate sleep.

It might interest you to know that in the late 1800s, people averaged nine and a half hours of sleep each night. By the early 1980s, Americans averaged only seven and a half hours of sleep. In the 1990s, the average dropped to a little less than seven hours. We are continuing on our stress-laden, downward trend.

People who deprive themselves of sleep often boast, "But I get so much more work done." But do they?

We cannot cheat our bodies—at least not forever. We all have individual, biological needs for a certain amount of sleep. A few people truly need only six hours and some need as many as nine. There is no one set amount.

We may try to cheat, but it is like borrowing money. Payback time eventually comes. We can live with lesser amounts of sleep and increasing amounts of caffeine, but one day our bodies rebel. They rebel by breaking down. We call that sickness. Or our bodies become involved in accidents or have emotional or mental problems. Some way and in some form, our bodies eventually get taken care of or they stop taking care of us.

If we want to live healthy lives, **REST** is crucial. We can help maximize our health and longevity by getting the right amount of sleep that our individual bodies need.

\* \* \*

Are we getting enough sleep? If we are not, we probably nod off whenever we are not active—sitting in church, or watching TV.

If we always need an alarm to awaken us, we're probably not providing for our biological sleep need.

If we sleep longer on our days off or on weekends it probably means we are not getting enough sleep the other nights.

The best way to find our how much sleep we need is to set aside one week, perhaps during vacation time, where we can spend up to nine hours in uninterrupted sleep. If we set no alarm clocks, we allow our bodies to adjust and set their own rhythm and the amount of sleep consistently needed.

"Listen to your body's wisdom," a friend said recently. "Your body may be giving you messages that your brain does not want to hear."

\* \* \*

Seventh-day Adventists have one practice that distinguishes them from most Christian denominations: their adherence to the fourth commandment: "Remember the Sabbath Day to keep it holy." (*Exodus 20:8 NIV*) They believe the proper observance of the Sabbath brings them physical and mental benefits.

This is the basic command to rest.

The root of the word **Sabbath** means "to stop, rest, cease." This refers to God's acts of creation. After bringing the world into being, God stopped, not from tiredness, but because he had finished his work. This is the reasoning behind the command to observe the seventh-day Sabbath. Adherents of this biblical principle believe that God intended them to "finish" their work for the week. They totally drop it.

The fourth commandment reads:

Remember the Sabbath day to keep it holy. Six days shalt thou labor and do all thy work, but the seventh day is the Sabbath of the LORD thy God. In it thou shalt not do any work, thou, nor thy son, nor thy daughter, thy manservant, nor thy maidservant, nor thy cattle, nor thy stranger that is within thy gates: For in six days the LORD made heaven and the earth, the sea, and all that in them is, and rested the seventh day: wherefore the LORD blessed the Sabbath day, and hallowed it (*Exodus 20:8-11 KJV.*)

Two parts comprise that command. First, you work six days. No excuse for idleness. Second, you rest the day. The rest follows the work. God wisely made that provision thousands of years ago.

We live in a fast-paced, stress-filled life. The idea of ceasing from work for an entire 24 hours sounds overwhelming to many.

Yet the Sabbath can become a special vacation-like day—a time to put aside our work, schedules, and daily commitments—once a week. We can rest, relax, refocus, and enjoy our Creator and each other. Following the ancient practice of the Old Testament, a strict observance of the Sabbath means to maintain the holy atmosphere from sundown Friday until sundown Saturday, a true 24-hour period.

This habitual one-day-out-of-seven rest provides a relatively stress-free environment and gives us an opportunity to respond to Jesus' words, "Come apart and rest." (Mark 6:31) On this day, seek solitude in the out-of-doors and avoid stress-producing noise. Avoid jammed freeways, shopping malls, packed stadiums, competitive sports, and you maintain healthier blood pressure levels.

When we say, "I do not have time for a day of rest every week," we are really saying, "I am too busy to obey God and too busy to take care of myself."

The Sabbath observance is a time to cease from work, but it is more. It is also time to cease from accomplishment, from worry and tension, and to stop trying to control our lives. This is important because we exist to live in a world where we constantly strive to make everything go our way. We can benefit most if we see this as a day set aside for physical rest and spiritual refreshment.

We also can think about **why** God gave that command. God sanctified (that is, set apart) the 7th day for the good of humanity. The people were to work for six days and then they were to rest for one—a rhythm that history has shown fits human life. If the command to rest one day out of seven is for the good of the human race, then ponder carefully the implications of saying "no" to this strong Old Testament command.

In the New Testament, Jesus said the Sabbath was made for humanity, not for humanity to slavishly follow a law. (*Mark 2:27.*) He also said that it was a day "to do good" (*Matthew 12:12*), to save (*Mark 3:4*), to free people from physical and spiritual bondage (*Luke 12:12*), and to show mercy (*Matthew 12:7*).

Above all, the 7th day is not just a day off from work. To think in such a way focuses on utilitarianism. Sabbath means stop and to move into a different kind of time. When we keep God's ordinance, it makes all our activities—participation in informal fellowship and recreation as well as participation in formal worship—offerings to God.

### T is for TRUST—Trust in the Lord

When we trust—believe—the Lord, it shows in our life, through our relationships with our families and the way we treat other people.

Trust in God brings joy, peace, and fulfillment, which nothing else can do. Even secular research is now affirming that all forms of spiritual belief and faith exert a powerful benefit to healthy living. Recent experiments have shown that patients who were prayed for in

179

hospitals recovered quicker than those who were not prayed for, even if they did not know about it.

Westerners are now learning the health benefits of faith in a loving God. They are opening themselves to praying, meditating, helping others, reading spiritual literature and are realizing that these activities mobilize us against disease.

On a national TV newscast one scientist said something like this: The body follows the mind's expectations. If we hold strong spiritual convictions they strengthen our inner forces that keep our minds calm and direct the hypothalamus gland to relax.

"If we believe in God and rely on a higher power, we now see that as the best of all possible methods for managing stress," said a stress-management expert in 1997 in Atlanta. "Belief in a higher power releases energies that provide values to live for and a purpose for living."

I can affirm that and speak from my own experience. I was dying and I turned to God. When I turned, God lovingly accepted me, healed me, and changed my life.

My story is not unique. In our denomination—and in others as well—we have thousands of testimonies that show a strong correlation between faith and improved health and longevity.

Faith in God gives us the spiritual rest, the inner assurance that God is in control of the world and of our lives. I heard about a study going on in Maryland a few years ago that compared church people with the general population. Men who were involved in their church and said they tried to live by helping others, had a heart disease rate of 50 percent below that of the local population. They also expressed less loneliness and had a higher self-image.

Faith, of course, comes from God. We can't make it happen, but we can open ourselves to God through prayer, reading the Bible, and being with other believers.

* * *

As I write this book, I can testify that I am alive today because of God's grace and help of others and my willingness to make changes in my life. I believe in God. My belief in God has made all the difference in the world.

## Esther's Reflections.....

To see Ben walk, then able to run and able to eat—brought tears of joy. Those tears, I did not hide from him. He knew I was very happy. But many times he had a hard time getting his food down. I took notes on what food was easily digested and what caused him to have pain. At that time, I decided to make choices for him because I just could not stand to see him suffering any more. I decided I would prepare and eat only food that he could tolerate. It worked at home. But not when we went to church for potlucks, or ate out.

Most of the time, massage, walking and hydrotherapy helped him a lot. It felt so good to hear and see him happy after coming out of the CAT Scan room cancer-free. There were many months filled with pain and sleepless nights, but they were also good times because we were always together.

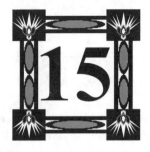

# I'm a Miracle

*"I was lost to the skills of men and bound to die*
*But because of Your plan for me,*
*You heard my cry.*
*And you came in response to prayer and eased my pain*
*So I won't live the rest of my life in vain.*
*I'm a miracle, Lord, because of you."*
—Dan Burgess

By 1997, I had gone on full medical disability. Occasionally I thought about going back to work, but most of my friends did not want to hear me talk that way. Amazed that I was alive and getting healthy, they did not think there was any possibility that I would ever get well enough to go back to my medical practice again.

I did not think so either.

But I often thought about it. I even prayed that God would make it possible. I would not say I believed it would happen, because I did not. I liked my new lifestyle, and I was alive and serving God. But still I missed my medical practice and working with sick people and other doctors.

I had things to do and I kept busy. Esther and I went together to different places in the US and foreign countries like the Marshall Islands, Indonesia, as well as to the Philippines, Singapore, Thailand and India. At each seminar, I stood before thousands of people and gave them the story of my recovery from terminal cancer. "Today I am alive. And because I am alive against all medical indications," I said, "I am a living miracle."

\* \* \*

My disability insurance required that I return every six months for a physical to certify the need to continue payments. In 1996, I had received the diagnosis of terminal cancer. In 1999, I was still alive—which astounded many. I went to the oncologist selected by the insurance company for an examination.

"I can't tell you the results," he said after he had checked me thoroughly. The insurance company had hired him, and he was responsible to give them his report. "I can tell you this much. You're 95 percent cured."

"Really?" I asked. I was surprised that he would say that. Except for my energy level that was not quite normal, I felt healthy and well. "When I come back next year, will I be 100 percent cured?"

He smiled, but he did not answer.

I had known I was getting better, and now—for the first time—I sensed that God might be directing me to go back to my medical practice. Because I believed that, I began to read the new literature, to attend medical seminars, and to become active again in the American Society of Anesthesiologists. If God provided the opportunity for me to return to work, I wanted to be ready.

In March 2000, I had my next CAT Scan. It was negative. After four years, I was still free of cancer.

"Amazing," was the response I heard from Dr. Purewal, my medical doctor.

"May I go back to work?" I asked. "I feel I am now able to work full time and take anesthesia calls again." It took a few days and a little paper work, before my doctor and the insurance company released me.

I had not practiced for four years. Yet I wanted to get back to work as quickly as possible.

One day before the end of March 2000, I approached Dr. Ila Madia, a practicing anesthesiologist. She knew my history, of course.

"I would love to come back to work again, doctor, do you have a place for me?"

"I am going to talk to my husband about it," she said.

To demonstrate my sincere desire, I wrote a letter of application to Dr. Dalsukh Madia. I told him that it would certainly be an honor to be employed by him in any capacity as an anesthesiologist.

Dr. Madia and his wife headed a group of active CRNAs (Certified Registered Nurse Anesthetist), and had practiced anesthesiology in Marion for more than 20 years.

They made a sensible arrangement with me. For a month, I was hired as a **locum tenem**—which is like working for the group by contract. They observed me and saw that I was physically fit and was able to do the work.

"We want to extend the invitation for you to join the group," Dr. Madia said.

I was overjoyed. It was so wonderful to be able to be back at work and doing what I had been trained to do.

I started with the group in May 2000. As required in the contract, it would take two years for me to earn the right to become a full partner.

At the time of this writing, I am not yet a full partner, but I am not worried. God has performed one miracle after another for me. They said I would not live more than a few months. But with God's help, a supportive wife and family, and caring friends, I am still alive. More than just being alive, I have triumphed over terminal cancer.

I am a miracle.

And each day I thank God.

---

## *Esther's Final Reflections.....*

Ben surprised me one day when he came home after attending a medical meeting at the Smith Clinic. That week we had discussed selling the house and moving into an apartment to simplify our lives. Sure, Ben acted and looked very healthy and strong. But he could not tolerate foods like broccoli, which he loved so much, and he felt pain after meals. The hydrotherapy and exercises helped, yet I always felt so sorry for him. And that is the reason that I wanted to sell the house: then we could have more time together and not worry about maintenance on the house and other financial obligations.

When he came home that day in early March, he excitedly told me there was a job opportunity for him...I had mixed feelings. I cannot explain why I gave him so much encouragement. I knew I would miss him after enjoying his company for almost 24 hours a day and sharing the traveling crusades. I was afraid that our lives would return to the same hectic routine we had before cancer. I also worried about how he would be able to do his routine treatment, how the stress of the work would affect him and his new eating habits, and if all this would enable the cancer to return. So many things went through my mind. Yet I also knew how much his work meant to him. So I resolved that I would find ways to support him: Like taking his meals to the hospital, reminding him to exercise and pray so he could handle his cases with confidence, and to stay out of the hospital's political problems.

Then of course we had concerns about how he would be accepted by patients and other doctors: "Is Ben alert enough? Is he capable of administering anesthesia after not practicing for almost five years? What if he gets sick while administering anesthetics?" We realized that if doctors had uneasy feelings towards him that Ben must understand. Sure enough, there were times when other doctors felt that he might not be capable of giving anesthesia to their patients. But I thank God that things worked out the way they should. The doctors and nurses have been very helpful to him. Above all, I am thankful that the Madias understand Ben's needs and support his participation in health lectures all over the world, where he is invited to share his story. Ben is now busy with his practice, but still finds time to accept invitations to speak at local health seminars sponsored by the American Cancer Society and Insurance companies, as well as, talking to other cancer patients from USA and Canada.

Though we have experienced so much pain and difficulty, at the same time we have found joy in serving our fellow humans and God. It is really a great joy for me that Ben can continue to do what the Lord wants him to do. I turn my eyes to Jesus, for I need Him every hour in my life. I know I have done everything that I can possibly do as Ben's wife, friend and private nurse. And the rest I give to Him...I give and surrender ALL.

Just writing about this makes me feel down. Remembering Ben's suffering makes me feel so sad. I never had an opportunity to grieve when it was all happening. So this is my opportunity now. Yes, the pain and trials made our family closer. They helped us understand each other better. And we drew even closer to God. We survived by having faith in God, by believing that what we asked for could happen, and then by working hard together to make it happen. And I am so glad and thankful that it worked. I know God will continue blessing us, and I will have many more years with Ben. I must quit writing now before I cry again—these tears of pain and joy. I also thank God for the MIRACLES!

# *Published Article "The Marion Star" May 2000*

By Darlene Slack

As Dr. Benjamin Sanidad slipped inside his green scrubs at Marion General Hospital April 5, it was like awakening from a long dream. Four years ago, he had been diagnosed with cancer of the esophagus. None of his colleagues would say it then, and he did not ask. "But," he said, "I saw it in their eyes: I'm a dead man."

Every esophageal cancer patient he knew had died within months. Usually, it is not diagnosed until advanced stages, and once spread beyond the esophagus (the tube that carries food to the stomach); there is no known cure. Sanidad, then 51 and an anesthesiologist, resigned to his fate. He accepted treatment because he understood a doctor's determination to do whatever possible, even when hope is dim.

But as he recovered from surgery that removed his esophagus and part of his stomach—the same surgery that revealed the cancer already had spread to his lymph nodes—Sanidad started to fight for the life and family he loved.

This spring, he celebrated an unexpected anniversary. "Instead of four more months, it's been four more years," he said. "And there's no trace of cancer."

More than one colleague has told him: "It's a miracle you're alive."

"We do a lot of hugging these days." Said Vickie McCleland, an MGH nurse, describing how it feels to see a friend with "a death sentence" well and working again with significant changes.

Gone is "the round cuddly guy we had known before," she said. Sanidad is still 5-foot 3 1/2 inches, but 50 pounds lighter, his weight loss now a sign of health rather than sickness. Simultaneously, he has "expanded" in other ways: a deeper calm and joy as he works, a deeper understanding of patients.

"He's always been an excellent physician, but unless you've experienced something life threatening and scary, you don't know how dependent patients are on (us)" she said. "Ben told me, `Now I look at my patients and I know the fears and the questions they're having.'"

Dr. Frederick Winegarner vividly remembers March 31, 1996, when he found cancer in his friend and colleague of 20 years. The day before, Sanidad collapsed at the end of a patient's surgery and that night passed blood in his stool. As Winegarner looked down an endo-scope, a flexible tube with light and video camera, into stomach, he expected to find an ulcer.

"When I saw the tumor my eyes filled with tears," he said. "It was hard to be an objective treating physician of someone I really cared about."

"It was a scary situation," said Sanidad's eldest son, Ben. "All the experiences we had came to mind—good and bad. The regrets, the negative stuff we had, and all the fun times. I tried not to focus on what it was going to be like if he was not around anymore."

Dr. Christopher Ellison, now acting Chairman at the Ohio State University Hospital surgery department in Columbus, removed the cancerous organs and some lymph nodes, then made a new esophagus from Sanidad's stomach. He recommended chemotherapy and radia-tion to destroy the remaining cancer cells. As he recovered from sur-gery, however, Sanidad researched his options. Nothing guaranteed a cure. But one treatment made more sense to him than others. A bit nervous, he told his doctors he wanted to try alternative medicine.

"Most of us felt like his case had a poor outlook regardless of whether he took chemotherapy or not," Winegarner said. But Sanidad, as both doctor and cancer patient, exercised "radical thinking to go the natural route rather than the conventional route. Most people in desperation will want to try anything that might work."

Sanidad and his wife, Esther, followed the "little ray of hope" that led to alternative medicine. To them, chemotherapy (drugs) and radiation (X-ray therapy) had too many undesirable side effects, such as damaging healthy cells with cancerous ones. They chose to fight the cancer naturally by increasing the body's immune system.

The biggest challenge would be the struggle within Dr. Sanidad. "With cancer you go through a stage of not caring if you live or die. Ben went through that," said Esther Sanidad, a former nurse. "You have to want to do it. You have to be willing to be alive."

Three months after his diagnosis, the Sanidads enrolled in an 18-day program at Hartland Wellness Center in Rapidan, VA, one of several centers established in the early 1980s to promote health through natural remedies. Because family support is recommended, the Sanidad's three adult children, Ben, Nikki, and Arti, eventually completed the program, too.

Through daily lecture and hands-on participation from cooking to massage, the Sanidads learned an alternative lifestyle called NEW-START: nutrition, exercise, water therapy, sunshine, temperance, air, rest, and trust in God.

The holistic approach tends body, mind and spirit. Carrot juice rids the body of toxins. Exercise releases endorphins, enhancing one's sense of well-being. Water therapy (extended hot bath, then cold) increases white blood cells to fight infection. Meditation and prayer provide a different perspective for handling stress.

As Sanidad's new esophagus adjusted, he practiced other simple, life-saving habits, like chewing well and slowly. Otherwise, food could get stuck, choking him or affecting his heart,

Ellison cautioned that the new esophagus eventually would restrict and have to be dilated. That never occurred. But a year and a half after his surgery, Sanidad almost died when his intestine twisted around the scar tissue where a feeding tube had been inserted.

He waited for a surgeon through seven hours of intense pain in an emergency room in Canada, where his parents live. Surgery revealed 60% of his intestine "black" and clinically dead. Sanidad saw the bright lights described in near-death experiences. But he also heard his wife's voice telling him not to give up.

As the surgeon applied hot packs and waited for the swelling to decrease so he could suture Sanidad's stomach, unexpectedly, the intestine started "to pink up." Esther Sanidad took her husband home for recovery because she knew how effective the support; love and prayers expressed at MGH had been in his recovery.

Sanidad eventually traveled with his wife, a concert manager for different Christian recording artists, to share his story of recovery and faith at Seventh-day Adventist crusades. Feeling somewhat like a leper, he was a reluctant public speaker at first. But his inspirational message prompted invitations to health seminars in Florida, California, Chicago, Canada, India, Indonesia, Thailand, Singapore and his homeland, the Philippines.

Stronger and healthier than before his cancer diagnosis, Sanidad believes, "God has given me another chance to prove my worth."

"Cancer is a funny thing. It can show up 20 years later." said Winegarner, who checks Sanidad every six months. "But as a scientist physician I would say Ben's chances of staying cured are pretty good. I just rejoice with him and his good health."

The day Sanidad returned to work, a former classmate of his son Ben, requested his services. As she awoke from the anesthetic, she told him, "Please do not get sick, again." Instead of me comforting her," Sanidad said, "She gave me the inspiration and self-confidence that I was seeking after four years of being out of the medical field."

# And That's The Power of Love!

By: Susan Loyer

(published at the Generally Speaking newsletter of MGH)

We've all heard the words—love conquers all, love lifts us up, as well as the millions of words used to say "I love you." But have you ever stopped to think about what those words really mean especially to the person you're saying them to? Well, Dr. Benjamin Sanidad Jr., over the past four years, has taken them all to heart and hung on to them as tightly as he can. From his family from his friends that love, and his faith in God, is what has gotten him through his ordeal with cancer.

When he left Marion General Hospital in 1996, having been a practicing anesthesiologist in our surgery department since 1975, there was not much hope by his friends here that he would ever return to work with them. And given his prognosis from that date, March 31, 1996, to where he is today, makes him truly a "walking miracle."

So when he walked into the surgery department at Marion General Hospital on May 1, 2000 to provide anesthesia for his first MGH surgery case since being diagnosed with cancer of the esophagus, what did it feel to him? And just how thrilled were his colleagues to see him return to practice?

Dr. Sanidad says he loves being back, back where he belongs! In the 20 years that preceded his illness, many close relationships had developed with the MGH staff. There were lots of hugs, and I'm sure, tears, the day Dr. Sanidad returned to his old friends. "We had learned to love each other, and just enjoy each other during that time. If I have tears, they are tears of happiness!" he says with his gentle smile. "There is such indescribable joy in my heart, every day that I wake up

191

and thank God for another day."

"Personally, Dr. Sanidad is inspiring," says Elaine Cilek, operating room RN. "Seeing someone who has been through this and has survived gives us all hope. He has always been a polite, friendly person and it's truly great to see him back. He's just so nice to work with."

Vickie McClellan, operating room RN, adds, "His priorities have changed since his illness and he is even more of a people doctor now than he was before. I often hear him say to a cancer patient that he knows how they feel, that he's been there too. It's just a miracle that he is back with us!"

"Dr. Sanidad and I got along very well before his illness," says Gary Prater, operating room RN. "And even though he was always kind to his patients, now he relates to them on the basis of personal experience. He is willing to share that experience with our cancer patients, giving them encouragement and hope."

"I don't know if he has any idea of how many of us were praying for him," says Jim Siverling, operating room RN, "but there were a lot of us. Even though we saw him periodically over the last several years, it is just so good to see him back to work!"

Dr. Sanidad admits that he had been "mentally" preparing himself for a year to return to work. A couple of weeks before returning to work, he was given the chance to observe and do hands-on cases under the supervision of Dr. Dalsukh Madia. And he has been amazed at how quickly his skills have returned to him, after being out of the medical environment for four years. But, one of the most important factors in his successful return to the job that he loves has been the genuine "welcome back" by the staff. "I consider every day that I have a 'bonus' day—I keep pinching myself to make sure I'm not in a dream!" Dr. Sanidad laughs. "And I am so happy to once again be working with friends and serving the Marion community."

THE END